# Chemotherapy

## A Patient's Guide to Treatment and Recovery

Ethan D. Anderson

Xspurts.com

**A New Zealand Designed Product**

# Other Versions Available

Why limit yourself to just one format?

This book is now available in physical, digital, and audiobook options.

Choose the way you love to read and dive into the story today. You won't regret it!

**Digital ISBN:** 9781776967674
**Physical ISBN:** 9781776967667
**Audio ISBN:**

To obtain a different format of this book at a discounted price, please get in touch with us at:

http://isbn.xspurts.com/

# Contents

# Have Questions / Comments?

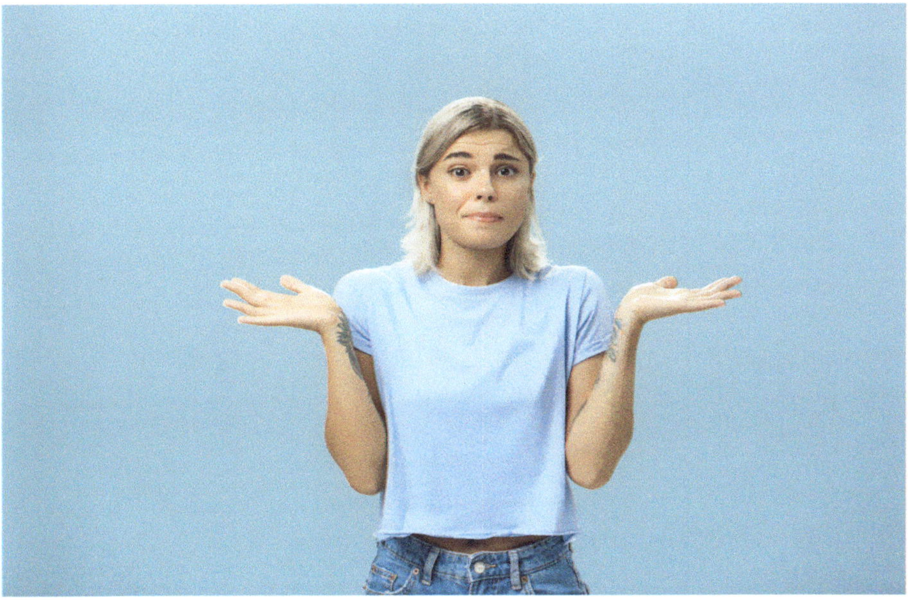

This book was designed to cover as much information as possible, but I know I have probably missed something, or some new amazing discovery has just come out.

If you notice something missing or have a question that I failed to answer, please get in touch and let me know. If I can, I will email you an answer and also update the book so others can also benefit from it.

Thanks For Being Awesome :)

**Submit Your Questions / Comments At:**

**https://questions.xspurts.com**

# Get Free Stuff

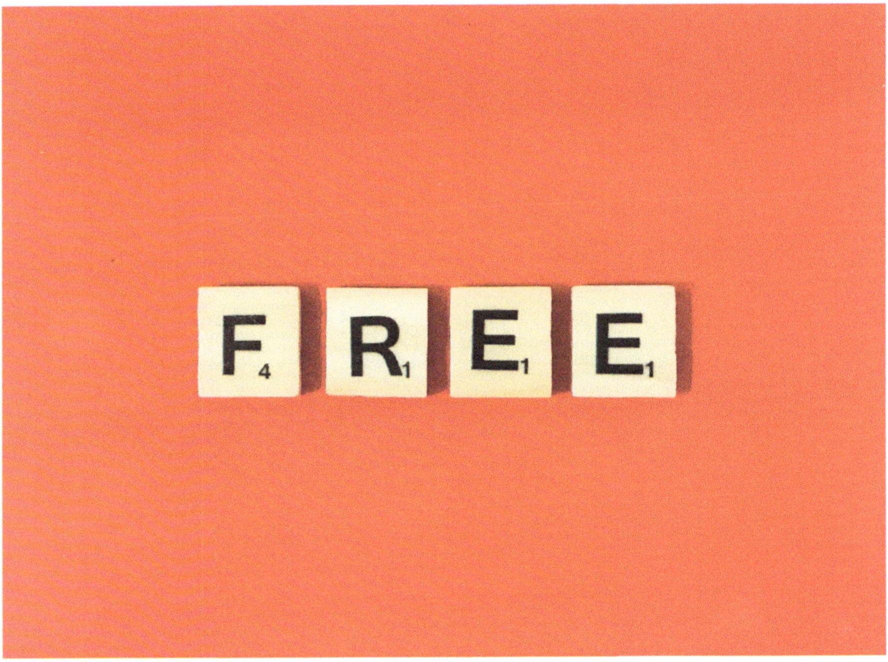


We love writing and have produced a huge number of books.

For being one of our amazing readers, we would love to offer you more books we have created, 100% free.

To claim this limited time special offer, simply go to the site below and enter your name and email address.

You will then receive loads (as we love our readers so much :) of our great books, content and audio direct to your email account, 100% free!

**Get Loads of FREE Stuff at:**

**https://free.xspurts.com**

Chapter One

# Understanding Chemotherapy: An Introduction

Chemotherapy is a widely recognized and commonly used treatment approach in the field of oncology. It plays a significant role in the management and treatment of various types of cancer. Chemotherapy utilizes powerful medications to target and destroy cancer cells, either by directly attacking them or by inhibiting their growth and division. This chapter aims to provide a comprehensive understanding of chemotherapy, its mechanisms of action, its side effects, and its role in cancer treatment.

Chemotherapy Basics

Chemotherapy is a systemic treatment, meaning it affects the entire body. It is designed to eliminate cancer cells wherever they may be present, including the primary tumor site and any potential metastatic sites. Unlike localized treatments, such as surgery or radiation therapy, chemotherapy is administered through various routes, including intravenous infusion, oral medications, or injections.

Mechanisms of Action

Chemotherapy drugs work through different mechanisms to combat cancer cells. Some drugs interfere with the DNA replication process, preventing cancer cells from dividing and proliferating. Others disrupt the cellular machinery necessary for cancer cell survival, ultimately leading to their death. Additionally, some chemotherapy drugs target specific proteins or receptors on the surface of cancer cells, inhibiting their growth signals and triggering cell death.

Types of Chemotherapy

Chemotherapy drugs can be categorized into different classes based on their chemical structure and mechanism of action. These classes include alkylating agents, antimetabolites, anthracyclines, taxanes, and platinum-based drugs, among others. The selection of specific chemotherapy drugs depends on several factors, such as the type and stage of cancer, the patient's overall health, and the potential side effects of the medications.

Combination Therapy

In many cases, chemotherapy drugs are administered in combination to maximize their effectiveness. Combining drugs with different mechanisms of action can enhance the treatment's overall impact by targeting cancer cells through multiple pathways. Combination chemotherapy also reduces the risk of drug resistance, as cancer cells are less likely to develop resistance to multiple drugs simultaneously.

Administration and Treatment Schedule

Chemotherapy can be administered in different cycles, depending on the treatment goals and the specific chemotherapy regimen. Treatment cycles typically consist of a period of active treatment, followed by a rest period to allow the body to recover from any potential side effects. The duration and frequency of treatment cycles vary, ranging from a few weeks to several months.

Side Effects of Chemotherapy

Chemotherapy affects both cancer cells and healthy cells, leading to a range of potential side effects. The most common side effects include fatigue, nausea and vomiting, hair loss, and a weakened immune system. However, it's important to note that not all patients experience the same side effects, and advancements in supportive care have significantly improved the management of chemotherapy-related side effects.

Personalized Approach

In recent years, there has been a shift towards a more personalized approach to chemotherapy. With advancements in molecular and genetic testing, oncologists can identify specific genetic mutations or biomarkers present in a patient's cancer cells. This information helps guide treatment decisions, allowing for targeted therapies that may be more effective and better tolerated.

Adjuvant and Neoadjuvant Chemotherapy

Chemotherapy is used in different settings within the cancer treatment journey. Adjuvant chemotherapy is administered after surgery or radiation therapy to eliminate any remaining cancer cells and reduce the risk of recurrence. Neoadjuvant chemotherapy, on the other hand, is given before surgery or radiation therapy to shrink tumors, making them more manageable for subsequent treatment.

Limitations and Future Directions

Although chemotherapy has proven to be an effective treatment option for many cancer types, it does have its limitations. Chemotherapy drugs can affect both healthy and cancerous cells, leading to various side effects. Furthermore, some cancers may develop resistance to certain chemotherapy drugs over time. As a result, ongoing research aims to develop more targeted

## The history of chemotherapy

Chemotherapy, as a cornerstone of cancer treatment, has a rich and fascinating history that spans several decades. The development of chemotherapy agents and the evolution of their use have revolutionized the field of oncology, leading to significant advancements in cancer care. This chapter explores the history of chemotherapy, highlighting key milestones, breakthroughs, and notable figures who have contributed to its development.

Early Beginnings

The origins of chemotherapy can be traced back to the early 20th century when researchers first observed the toxic effects of certain chemicals on rapidly dividing cells. In the 1940s, during World War II, researchers investigating the effects of mustard gas exposure on soldiers discovered that it not only caused harm but also affected cancer cells. This realization laid the foundation for the development of the first chemotherapy agents.

Milestone Discoveries

In the 1940s and 1950s, pioneering scientists made significant breakthroughs in chemotherapy research. One notable milestone was the discovery of the anti-cancer properties of the compound nitrogen mustard, leading to the development of the first chemotherapy drug, mechlorethamine. This discovery marked the beginning of a new era in cancer treatment.

In the subsequent years, researchers discovered other chemotherapy agents, including antimetabolites like methotrexate and antimicrotubule agents like vincristine. These discoveries were driven by a better understanding of cancer cell biology and the development of screening methods to identify compounds with anti-cancer properties.

Combination Chemotherapy

During the 1960s and 1970s, the concept of combination chemotherapy emerged. Researchers found that using multiple chemotherapy drugs in combination could improve treatment outcomes by targeting cancer cells through different mechanisms. Combination chemotherapy became a standard practice for many cancers, leading to increased cure rates and improved survival rates.

The Birth of Targeted Therapy

The late 20th century witnessed a shift towards more targeted approaches in cancer treatment. Scientists discovered specific cellular targets and signaling pathways that played a crucial role in cancer cell growth and survival. This knowledge paved the way for the development of targeted therapies, which selectively inhibit these targets, sparing healthy cells and reducing side effects.

One notable example is the introduction of imatinib, a tyrosine kinase inhibitor, in the early 2000s. Imatinib revolutionized the treatment of chronic myeloid leukemia (CML) by specifically targeting the abnormal protein produced by the Philadelphia chromosome, which drives the growth of CML cells. This breakthrough marked a significant milestone in the era of personalized medicine.

Advancements in Supportive Care

Throughout the history of chemotherapy, significant advancements have been made in supportive care. Early chemotherapy treatments were associated with severe side effects and limited supportive measures. However, over time, researchers developed strategies to manage and minimize these side effects, greatly improving the quality of life for patients undergoing chemotherapy.

Supportive care measures include the use of antiemetic medications to control nausea and vomiting, blood transfusions to manage anemia, growth factors to boost the production of white blood cells, and improved pain management techniques. These advancements have played a vital role in enhancing patient tolerance and compliance with chemotherapy regimens.

Ongoing Research and Future Directions

Despite the remarkable progress in chemotherapy, challenges remain. Some cancers develop resistance to chemotherapy drugs, and certain types of cancer still have limited treatment options. Researchers are actively investigating novel agents, combination strategies, and immunotherapies to overcome these challenges and improve treatment outcomes.

Personalized medicine is a rapidly advancing field within chemotherapy, aiming to tailor treatments based on an individual's genetic profile, tumor characteristics, and other factors. Advances in molecular testing, genomics, and proteomics have paved the way for precision oncology, where treatment decisions are guided by the unique features of each patient's cancer.

Moreover, researchers are exploring innovative delivery methods to improve

## How chemotherapy works

Chemotherapy is a powerful and widely used treatment modality in the field of oncology. It employs the use of medications to combat cancer cells and inhibit their growth. Understanding how chemotherapy works is key to appreciating its impact on cancer treatment. This chapter explores the mechanisms of action of chemotherapy, highlighting its effects on cancer cells and the challenges it presents.

### Halting Cell Division

One of the primary mechanisms of chemotherapy is the disruption of cell division. Cancer cells proliferate rapidly, dividing at a much higher rate than normal cells. Chemotherapy drugs target this rapid division by interfering with the DNA replication process, preventing cancer cells from dividing and multiplying.

Different chemotherapy drugs act on various stages of the cell cycle. Some drugs, known as cell-cycle-specific agents, are effective during specific phases of cell division. Others, referred to as cell-cycle non-specific agents, can act on cancer cells at any point in the cell cycle. The combination of these drugs helps to ensure that cancer cells are targeted effectively.

### Attacking DNA and RNA

Chemotherapy drugs exert their effects by damaging the DNA or RNA within cancer cells. They can either directly bind to the DNA or RNA, preventing them from functioning properly, or they can induce chemical changes within these molecules, leading to errors during cell replication.

For example, alkylating agents, such as cyclophosphamide, add alkyl groups to the DNA, causing cross-linking between DNA strands and preventing proper replication. Similarly, antimetabolites, like methotrexate, mimic essential components of DNA or RNA, leading to faulty replication or inhibiting the production of nucleotides necessary for cell division.

### Triggering Cell Death

Another important mechanism of chemotherapy is the induction of cell death, particularly programmed cell death or apoptosis. Apoptosis is a natural process in which cells self-destruct to maintain a healthy balance in the body. Cancer cells often have defective apoptotic mechanisms, allowing them to survive and multiply. Chemotherapy drugs can trigger apoptosis, causing cancer cells to undergo programmed cell death.

By targeting cancer cells and activating apoptotic pathways, chemotherapy drugs aim to eliminate these abnormal cells from the body. This mechanism is particularly important in treating cancers that are resistant to other treatment modalities, such as radiation therapy or surgery.

Inhibiting Blood Vessel Formation

Cancer cells require a blood supply to grow and spread. Without adequate oxygen and nutrients, cancer cells cannot survive and thrive. Chemotherapy drugs can target the process of angiogenesis, which is the formation of new blood vessels, thereby inhibiting the cancer's ability to establish a blood supply.

Anti-angiogenic chemotherapy agents, like bevacizumab, work by blocking the signals that promote blood vessel formation. This deprives cancer cells of the necessary resources for growth and can slow down or inhibit tumor progression.

Targeting Specific Molecular Pathways

Advances in cancer research have led to the development of targeted therapies, which aim to exploit specific molecular abnormalities in cancer cells. These targeted chemotherapy drugs focus on specific molecular pathways that are essential for cancer cell survival and growth.

For instance, tyrosine kinase inhibitors (TKIs) target specific enzymes that play a critical role in cancer cell signaling. TKIs, such as imatinib, bind to these enzymes and inhibit their activity, interrupting the signals that promote cancer cell growth and proliferation. Targeted chemotherapy allows for more precise and selective treatment, sparing healthy cells and reducing side effects.

Combination Therapy

Combination chemotherapy, the use of multiple chemotherapy drugs simultaneously, is a common approach in cancer treatment. This strategy aims to enhance treatment efficacy and overcome drug resistance. By combining drugs with different mechanisms of action, combination chemotherapy targets cancer cells through multiple pathways, reducing the likelihood of cancer cells developing resistance to treatment.

Additionally, combination chemotherapy can target cancer cells at

Chapter Two

# Types of Chemotherapy Drugs

Chemotherapy drugs form the backbone of cancer treatment, with numerous types available to target different cancer types and stages. These drugs vary in their mechanisms of action and side effects, allowing oncologists to tailor treatment regimens to individual patients. Understanding the different types of chemotherapy drugs is crucial in comprehending their diverse effects on cancer cells. This chapter explores several categories of chemotherapy drugs, highlighting their characteristics and applications.

Alkylating Agents:

Alkylating agents are among the oldest and most commonly used chemotherapy drugs. They work by directly damaging the DNA within cancer cells, inhibiting their ability to replicate and divide. Examples of alkylating agents include cyclophosphamide, cisplatin, and temozolomide. These drugs are effective against various cancers, including leukemia, lymphoma, and solid tumors.

Antimetabolites:

Antimetabolites interfere with the production of essential molecules required for DNA and RNA synthesis, impeding cancer cell division. They mimic the structure of nucleotides, inhibiting their incorporation into DNA during replication. Methotrexate, fluorouracil, and cytarabine are common antimetabolites used to treat cancers such as breast, colon, and leukemia.

Anthracyclines:

Anthracyclines are potent chemotherapy drugs derived from Streptomyces bacteria. They work by intercalating with DNA, disrupting replication, and inducing DNA damage. Additionally, anthracyclines can generate reactive oxygen species, leading to further DNA destruction. Commonly used anthracyclines include doxorubicin and daunorubicin, employed in the treatment of breast cancer, lymphomas, and other solid tumors.

Taxanes:

Taxanes, derived from the bark of the Pacific yew tree, exert their effects by inhibiting microtubule assembly, a vital component of cell division. By stabilizing microtubules, taxanes prevent their breakdown during mitosis, leading to cell cycle arrest and apoptosis. Paclitaxel and docetaxel are widely used taxanes in the treatment of breast, lung, and ovarian cancers.

Platinum-Based Drugs:

Platinum-based drugs, including cisplatin and carboplatin, form covalent bonds with DNA, causing cross-linking between strands and interfering with DNA repair mechanisms. This disruption inhibits cancer cell replication and triggers apoptosis. Platinum-based drugs are used in the treatment of various solid tumors, such as testicular, ovarian, and lung cancers.

Topoisomerase Inhibitors:

1. Topoisomerase inhibitors target enzymes known as topoisomerases, which control the structure and integrity of DNA during replication. By interfering with these enzymes, topoisomerase inhibitors impede DNA unwinding and repair, resulting in DNA damage and cell death. Topoi-

somerase inhibitors are categorized into two types: topoisomerase I inhibitors (e.g., irinotecan) and topoisomerase II inhibitors (e.g., etoposide). These drugs are used in the treatment of leukemia, lung, and gastrointestinal cancers.

Hormonal Agents:

Hormonal agents are specific to hormone receptor-positive cancers, such as breast and prostate cancers. These drugs target the hormone receptors on cancer cells and inhibit their ability to receive hormone signals, which contribute to cancer growth. Examples include tamoxifen, used in hormone receptor-positive breast cancer, and leuprolide, employed in prostate cancer treatment.

Immunomodulatory Drugs:

Immunomodulatory drugs, such as thalidomide and lenalidomide, stimulate the body's immune system to recognize and attack cancer cells. They modify the tumor microenvironment and enhance immune responses against cancer

## Alkylating agents

Chemotherapy, a cornerstone of cancer treatment, encompasses a diverse range of drugs with distinct mechanisms of action. Among these drugs, alkylating agents play a crucial role in combating cancer cells. Alkylating agents are a class of chemotherapy drugs that directly damage the DNA within cancer cells, impairing their ability to replicate and divide. This chapter delves into the fascinating world of alkylating agents, exploring their mechanisms of action, common examples, and applications in cancer treatment.

Mechanism of Action

Alkylating agents exert their effects by forming covalent bonds with the DNA molecule, leading to the disruption of DNA structure and function. These drugs contain chemically reactive alkyl groups that transfer to DNA, causing DNA cross-linking, single-strand breaks, or DNA adduct formation. By inducing such DNA damage, alkylating agents impede the replication and transcription processes, ultimately resulting in cell cycle arrest and apoptosis.

Types of Alkylating Agents

Alkylating agents encompass a wide range of compounds with diverse chemical structures and properties. Some common examples include:

Cyclophosphamide:

Cyclophosphamide is one of the most widely used alkylating agents. It is a prodrug that requires activation by liver enzymes to form its active metabolite, phosphoramide mustard. This metabolite forms cross-links within DNA strands, preventing their separation and inhibiting DNA replication. Cyclophosphamide is employed in the treatment of various cancers, including leukemia, lymphoma, breast, and ovarian cancers.

Cisplatin:

Cisplatin is a platinum-based alkylating agent known for its remarkable efficacy against several solid tumors. It forms covalent bonds with DNA, leading to the formation of intrastrand and interstrand cross-links. These cross-links distort the DNA helix, impeding replication and transcription. Cisplatin is commonly used in the treatment of testicular, ovarian, and bladder cancers.

Carmustine:

Carmustine, also known as BCNU, is an alkylating agent belonging to the nitrosourea class. It readily crosses the blood-brain barrier, making it particularly effective against brain tumors. Carmustine alkylates DNA at the O^6-guanine position, leading to the formation of DNA adducts and subsequent DNA strand breaks. It is used in the treatment of brain tumors, lymphomas, and multiple myeloma.

Mechlorethamine:

Mechlorethamine, the earliest developed alkylating agent, is used primarily in the treatment of Hodgkin's lymphoma and other lymphomas. It directly attacks DNA by alkylating the guanine base, causing DNA cross-linking and DNA strand breaks. Mechlorethamine is typically administered topically or intravenously due to its potent vesicant properties.

Applications in Cancer Treatment

Alkylating agents find widespread use in the treatment of various cancers due to their broad-spectrum activity and ability to target rapidly dividing cells. They are employed in different settings, including:

Curative Treatment:

Alkylating agents are often part of curative treatment regimens, particularly for hematological malignancies like leukemia and lymphoma. These drugs are included in combination chemotherapy protocols, targeting cancer cells at different stages of the cell cycle and improving treatment efficacy.

Adjuvant Therapy:

Alkylating agents are frequently utilized as adjuvant therapy, administered after surgery or radiation therapy, to eradicate any remaining cancer cells and reduce the risk of recurrence. By attacking residual cancer cells, adjuvant chemotherapy can help improve long-term outcomes.

Palliative Treatment:

In cases where a

## Antimetabolites

Chemotherapy, a vital component of cancer treatment, encompasses a diverse array of drugs with distinct mechanisms of action. Among these drugs, antimetabolites stand out as key players in the fight against cancer. Antimetabolites are a class of chemotherapy drugs that disrupt cancer cell growth by interfering with the production of essential molecules required for DNA and RNA synthesis. This chapter delves into the intriguing world of antimetabolites, exploring their mechanisms of action, common examples, and applications in cancer treatment.

Mechanism of Action

Antimetabolites exert their effects by masquerading as natural molecules required for DNA and RNA synthesis, thereby disrupting the normal metabolic processes within cancer cells. They are structural analogs or synthetic substitutes that resemble nucleotides, the building blocks of DNA and RNA. Once incorporated into the cellular machinery, antimetabolites interfere with key enzymes and processes involved in nucleotide synthesis, DNA replication, and RNA production. By doing so, they hinder the cancer cell's ability to divide, replicate, and carry out essential functions, ultimately leading to cell death.

Types of Antimetabolites

Antimetabolites encompass a variety of compounds with distinct structures and mechanisms of action. Some common examples include:

Methotrexate:

Methotrexate is a classic antimetabolite used in the treatment of various cancers, including breast, lung, and leukemias. It inhibits the enzyme dihydrofolate reductase, which is essential for the synthesis of tetrahydrofolate, a key coenzyme involved in nucleotide synthesis. By blocking this enzyme, methotrexate depletes the cell of essential precursors required for DNA and RNA synthesis, thereby impeding cancer cell growth.

Fluorouracil:

Fluorouracil, also known as 5-FU, is a fluorinated pyrimidine analog that disrupts DNA and RNA synthesis. It inhibits the enzyme thymidylate synthase, blocking the production of thymidine, a key component of DNA. Additionally, fluorouracil incorporates into RNA, leading to faulty RNA synthesis. By interfering with these processes, fluorouracil effectively hampers cancer cell proliferation. It is used to treat a wide range of cancers, including colorectal, breast, and gastrointestinal cancers.

Cytarabine:

Cytarabine, also referred to as cytosine arabinoside or ara-C, is a nucleoside analog that inhibits DNA synthesis. It is incorporated into the DNA molecule during replication, causing chain termination and preventing further DNA elongation. Cytarabine is primarily used in the treatment of acute myeloid leukemia (AML) and acute lymphoblastic leukemia (ALL).

Gemcitabine:

Gemcitabine is a nucleoside analog that disrupts both DNA and RNA synthesis. It is converted into its active form within the cell, where it competes with natural nucleotides for incorporation into growing DNA chains. Once incorporated, gemcitabine inhibits further DNA elongation and induces DNA strand termination. Additionally, gemcitabine interferes with RNA production, further impeding cancer cell proliferation. It is commonly used in the treatment of pancreatic, lung, and bladder cancers.

Applications in Cancer Treatment

Antimetabolites find extensive use in the treatment of various cancers due to their ability to target rapidly dividing cancer cells. They are employed in different settings, including:

Curative Treatment:

Antimetabolites are often employed as part of curative treatment regimens, particularly for leukemias, lymphomas, and solid tumors. They are typically

## Antitumor antibiotics

Chemotherapy, a vital component of cancer treatment, encompasses a diverse array of drugs with distinct mechanisms of action. Among these drugs, antitumor antibiotics stand out as potent weapons in the fight against cancer. Antitumor antibiotics are a class of chemotherapy drugs derived from natural sources, such as bacteria and fungi. They possess remarkable abilities to target cancer cells and inhibit their growth. This chapter delves into the intriguing world of antitumor antibiotics, exploring their mechanisms of action, common examples, and applications in cancer treatment.

Mechanism of Action

Antitumor antibiotics exert their effects by interfering with the vital processes of DNA replication and cell division. These drugs work by binding to DNA and inhibiting the activity of enzymes called topoisomerases, which are responsible for untangling and rearranging DNA during replication. By interfering with topoisomerases, antitumor antibiotics disrupt the normal functioning of DNA, preventing proper replication and leading to DNA damage. This disruption ultimately results in the inhibition of cancer cell growth and division.

Types of Antitumor Antibiotics

Antitumor antibiotics encompass a variety of compounds derived from natural sources. Some common examples include:

Doxorubicin:

Doxorubicin is one of the most widely used and effective antitumor antibiotics. It is derived from the bacterium Streptomyces peucetius var. caesius. Doxorubicin intercalates with DNA, inserting itself between DNA base pairs and interfering with DNA replication and transcription. Additionally, doxorubicin generates reactive oxygen species, which cause further DNA damage and cell death. This versatile drug is employed in the treatment of a wide range of cancers, including breast, lung, and ovarian cancers.

Daunorubicin:

Daunorubicin, also derived from Streptomyces bacteria, shares similarities with doxorubicin in terms of its mechanism of action. It intercalates with DNA, disrupting its structure and preventing normal replication and transcription. Daunorubicin is commonly used in the treatment of acute leukemias, particularly acute myeloid leukemia (AML).

Bleomycin:

Bleomycin is a unique antitumor antibiotic derived from Streptomyces verticillus. Unlike other antitumor antibiotics, bleomycin does not directly interfere with DNA replication. Instead, it induces DNA strand breaks by generating free radicals that cause oxidative damage to DNA. This oxidative damage leads to DNA breakage and inhibition of DNA synthesis. Bleomycin is primarily used in the treatment of testicular cancer, Hodgkin's lymphoma, and squamous cell carcinomas.

Mitomycin C:

Mitomycin C is a compound derived from Streptomyces bacteria. It possesses a unique mechanism of action, as it is not directly cytotoxic. Instead, mitomycin C is activated within the cell, forming cross-links between DNA strands and inhibiting DNA replication. Mitomycin C is commonly used in the treatment of various cancers, including bladder, stomach, and pancreatic cancers.

Applications in Cancer Treatment

Antitumor antibiotics find extensive use in the treatment of various cancers due to their potent effects on cancer cells. They are employed in different settings, including:

Curative Treatment:

Antitumor antibiotics are often used as part of curative treatment regimens for a variety of cancers. They are incorporated into combination chemotherapy protocols, targeting cancer cells at different stages of the cell cycle and improving treatment efficacy. These drugs play a crucial role in the eradication of cancer cells and the prevention of recurrence.

Combination Therapy:

Antitumor antibiotics are frequently used in combination with other chemotherapy drugs or treatment modalities to maximize their effectiveness. Combination chemotherapy

## Topoisomerase inhibitors

Chemotherapy, a vital component of cancer treatment, encompasses a diverse array of drugs with distinct mechanisms of action. Among these drugs, topoisomerase inhibitors stand out as crucial players in the fight against cancer. Topoisomerase inhibitors are a class of chemotherapy drugs that target the enzymes called topoisomerases, which play a pivotal role in DNA replication and transcription. By interfering with these enzymes, topoisomerase inhibitors disrupt the normal functioning of DNA and impede cancer cell growth. This chapter delves into the intriguing world of topoisomerase inhibitors, exploring their mechanisms of action, common examples, and applications in cancer treatment.

Mechanism of Action

2. Topoisomerases are essential enzymes that regulate the structure and integrity of DNA during replication and transcription. They work by temporarily breaking and rejoining DNA strands, relieving the tension and preventing the formation of knots or tangles in the DNA molecule. There are two types of topoisomerases: topoisomerase I and topoisomerase II.

Topoisomerase inhibitors disrupt the activity of these enzymes, leading to DNA damage and cell death. They either inhibit the ability of topoisomerases to break DNA strands (topoisomerase I inhibitors) or interfere with their ability to rejoin DNA strands (topoisomerase II inhibitors). By disrupting the proper functioning of topoisomerases, these inhibitors prevent the completion of DNA replication or transcription, ultimately leading to the inhibition of cancer cell growth.

Types of Topoisomerase Inhibitors

Topoisomerase inhibitors encompass a variety of compounds with distinct structures and mechanisms of action. Some common examples include:

Topoisomerase I Inhibitors:

Topoisomerase I inhibitors, as the name suggests, specifically target topoisomerase I. These inhibitors bind to the topoisomerase I-DNA complex, preventing the rejoining of DNA strands and causing DNA breaks. As a result, the replication and transcription processes are disrupted, leading to cancer cell death. Examples of topoisomerase I inhibitors include irinotecan and topotecan, which are used in the treatment of colorectal, lung, and ovarian cancers.

Topoisomerase II Inhibitors:

Topoisomerase II inhibitors target topoisomerase II and interfere with its ability to rejoin DNA strands. These inhibitors stabilize the topoisomerase II-DNA complex, leading to the formation of DNA breaks and the accumulation of double-strand breaks. By inhibiting the repair of DNA breaks, topoisomerase II inhibitors induce cell cycle arrest and apoptosis in cancer cells. Examples of topoisomerase II inhibitors include etoposide and doxorubicin, which are employed in the treatment of various cancers, including leukemia, lymphoma, and lung cancer.

Applications in Cancer Treatment

Topoisomerase inhibitors find extensive use in the treatment of various cancers due to their potent effects on cancer cells. They are employed in different settings, including:

Curative Treatment:

Topoisomerase inhibitors are often utilized as part of curative treatment regimens for different types of cancers. They are incorporated into combination chemotherapy protocols, targeting cancer cells at different stages of the cell cycle and improving treatment efficacy. These drugs play a crucial role in eradicating cancer cells and preventing recurrence.

Combination Therapy:

Topoisomerase inhibitors are frequently used in combination with other chemotherapy drugs or treatment modalities to maximize their effectiveness. Combination chemotherapy regimens, including topoisomerase inhibitors, are designed to enhance treatment outcomes by attacking cancer cells through multiple pathways. The synergistic effects of combination therapy can increase response rates and improve long-term survival.

Palliative Treatment:

Topoisom

## Mitotic inhibitors

Chemotherapy, a vital component of cancer treatment, encompasses a diverse array of drugs with distinct mechanisms of action. Among these drugs, mitotic inhibitors stand out as key players in the fight against cancer. Mitotic inhibitors are a class of chemotherapy drugs that specifically target the process of cell division, known as mitosis. By disrupting mitosis, these inhibitors impede cancer cell growth and division. This chapter delves into the intriguing world of mitotic inhibitors, exploring their mechanisms of action, common examples, and applications in cancer treatment.

Mechanism of Action

Mitotic inhibitors disrupt the normal progression of the cell cycle, specifically targeting the process of mitosis, during which cells divide and multiply. They interfere with the crucial steps of mitosis, preventing proper chromosome segregation and cell division. By doing so, mitotic inhibitors halt the proliferation of cancer cells, leading to their eventual death.

Types of Mitotic Inhibitors

Mitotic inhibitors encompass a variety of compounds with distinct structures and mechanisms of action. Some common examples include:

Vinca Alkaloids:

Vinca alkaloids, such as vinblastine and vincristine, are derived from the periwinkle plant. They inhibit microtubule formation, a critical process for mitosis. Vinca alkaloids bind to tubulin, a protein that makes up microtubules, and prevent their proper assembly. As a result, the mitotic spindle, which is essential for chromosome segregation, cannot form correctly, leading to cell cycle arrest and apoptosis. Vinca alkaloids are used in the treatment of various cancers, including leukemia, lymphoma, and breast cancer.

Taxanes:

Taxanes, including paclitaxel and docetaxel, are derived from the bark of the Pacific yew tree. They work by stabilizing microtubules, preventing their disassembly during mitosis. By stabilizing microtubules, taxanes impair the normal function of the mitotic spindle, preventing proper chromosome segregation and cell division. Taxanes are commonly used in the treatment of breast, ovarian, and lung cancers.

Epothilones:

Epothilones, such as ixabepilone, are a newer class of mitotic inhibitors that share similar mechanisms of action with taxanes. They also stabilize microtubules, preventing their disassembly during mitosis. Epothilones offer an alternative treatment option for patients who may have developed resistance to taxane-based chemotherapy. Ixabepilone is used in the treatment of breast cancer.

Applications in Cancer Treatment

Mitotic inhibitors find extensive use in the treatment of various cancers due to their potent effects on cancer cells. They are employed in different settings, including:

Curative Treatment:

Mitotic inhibitors are often utilized as part of curative treatment regimens for different types of cancers. They are incorporated into combination chemotherapy protocols, targeting cancer cells at different stages of the cell cycle and improving treatment efficacy. These drugs play a crucial role in eradicating cancer cells and preventing recurrence.

Combination Therapy:

Mitotic inhibitors are frequently used in combination with other chemotherapy drugs or treatment modalities to maximize their effectiveness. Combination chemotherapy regimens, including mitotic inhibitors, are designed to enhance treatment outcomes by attacking cancer cells through multiple pathways. The synergistic effects of combination therapy can increase response rates and improve long-term survival.

Palliative Treatment:

Mitotic inhibitors are also employed as palliative treatment to relieve symptoms and improve the quality of life for patients with advanced or metastatic cancers. These drugs can help shrink tumors, alleviate pain, and reduce cancer-related complications, leading to improved symptom control and overall well-being.

Neoad

Chapter Three

# Chemotherapy Treatment Plans

Chemotherapy is a powerful treatment modality in the fight against cancer. It encompasses a diverse range of drugs and treatment protocols tailored to individual patients and their specific cancer types. Developing a chemotherapy treatment plan involves careful consideration of various factors, including cancer stage, patient characteristics, and treatment goals. This chapter explores the intricacies of chemotherapy treatment plans, highlighting the key considerations, common strategies, and the evolving landscape of personalized medicine.

Individualizing Treatment Plans

Chemotherapy treatment plans are highly individualized, taking into account several factors unique to each patient. These factors include:

Cancer Type and Stage:

The specific type and stage of cancer play a crucial role in determining the appropriate chemotherapy regimen. Different cancers respond differently to various drugs, and the extent of disease progression guides the intensity and duration of treatment. Chemotherapy treatment plans are tailored to target the specific characteristics and vulnerabilities of each cancer type.

Patient Characteristics:

Patient characteristics, such as age, overall health, organ function, and presence of comorbidities, are taken into consideration when designing a treatment plan. Some chemotherapy drugs may have specific toxicity profiles or interactions with pre-existing conditions, necessitating adjustments to the treatment regimen to ensure patient safety and tolerability.

Treatment Goals:

The goals of chemotherapy treatment can vary depending on the individual case. The primary goal is often curative, aiming to eradicate the cancer and prevent its recurrence. In other cases, the goal may be palliative, focusing on symptom relief, improvement in quality of life, or slowing disease progression. Treatment plans are developed in alignment with the specific goals of therapy.

Common Strategies in Chemotherapy Treatment Plans

Chemotherapy treatment plans encompass various strategies to maximize treatment efficacy and minimize side effects. Some common strategies include:

Combination Chemotherapy:

Combination chemotherapy involves the use of multiple chemotherapy drugs in a coordinated treatment regimen. This strategy aims to attack cancer cells through different mechanisms, reducing the likelihood of drug resistance and improving treatment outcomes. Combination chemotherapy can also allow for lower doses of individual drugs, minimizing toxicities while maintaining effectiveness.

Neoadjuvant and Adjuvant Therapy:

Neoadjuvant chemotherapy refers to treatment given before surgery or radiation therapy. It aims to shrink tumors, making them more amenable to surgical resection or other local treatments. Adjuvant chemotherapy, on the other hand, is administered after surgery or radiation therapy to eliminate any remaining cancer cells and reduce the risk of recurrence. Neoadjuvant and adjuvant therapies are commonly employed in the treatment of breast, lung, and colorectal cancers, among others.

Dose Intensity and Schedule:

Dose intensity and treatment schedule are carefully considered in chemotherapy treatment plans. The dose intensity refers to the frequency and amount of drug administered over a given period. Higher dose intensity may be appropriate for certain aggressive cancers, while lower dose intensity may be chosen to minimize side effects in more vulnerable patients. The treatment schedule, including the interval between treatment cycles, is designed to balance effectiveness and tolerability.

Targeted Therapy:

Advances in molecular biology and genetics have led to the emergence of targeted therapy, which aims to inhibit specific molecular targets involved in cancer growth and progression. Targeted therapy drugs are often combined with traditional chemotherapy agents to enhance treatment effectiveness. Targeted therapies are tailored to individual patients based on the genetic characteristics of their cancer, allowing for a more precise and personalized approach to treatment.

Personalized Medicine and Chemotherapy

The field of chemotherapy is advancing rapidly, embracing the concept of personalized medicine. Personalized medicine involves tailoring treatment plans to the unique genetic, molecular, and clinical characteristics of individual patients and their tumors. This approach utilizes genomic profiling, biomarkers, and other diagnostic tools to identify specific targets and match patients with the most effective treatment

## Personalized treatment plans

Chemotherapy has long been a cornerstone of cancer treatment, but the field is rapidly evolving with the advent of personalized medicine. Personalized treatment plans harness the power of precision by tailoring therapy to the individual characteristics of patients and their specific cancer types. By integrating genomic profiling, biomarkers, and other diagnostic tools, personalized treatment plans offer the potential for more effective, targeted, and tailored approaches to chemotherapy. This chapter explores the concept of personalized treatment plans, highlighting their significance, key elements, and advancements in the field.

Understanding Personalized Treatment Plans

Personalized treatment plans, also known as precision medicine or targeted therapy, aim to optimize treatment outcomes by customizing therapy to each patient's unique characteristics. These plans leverage comprehensive patient profiling, including genetic information, molecular analysis, and clinical data, to guide treatment decisions. By identifying specific genetic mutations, biomarkers, or molecular alterations driving the growth of a patient's tumor, personalized treatment plans can select therapies that target these specific vulnerabilities, leading to more effective treatment strategies.

Key Elements of Personalized Treatment Plans

Genomic Profiling:

Genomic profiling involves analyzing a patient's tumor DNA to identify specific genetic alterations that may drive cancer growth. Techniques like next-generation sequencing (NGS) can identify mutations, gene amplifications, or fusions that can be targeted by specific drugs. Genomic profiling provides crucial information about a patient's tumor biology and helps guide treatment decisions in personalized treatment plans.

Biomarker Analysis:

Biomarkers are measurable indicators that reflect biological processes or characteristics associated with a disease. In personalized treatment plans, biomarker analysis helps identify specific markers that can predict treatment response or guide therapeutic choices. For example, the presence of a specific biomarker may indicate sensitivity to a particular chemotherapy drug, allowing for a more targeted approach.

Molecular Signatures:

Molecular signatures are patterns of gene expression or molecular alterations that provide insights into the behavior of tumors. Through techniques like gene expression profiling or proteomic analysis, molecular signatures can classify tumors into subtypes with distinct characteristics and responses to treatment. These signatures assist in selecting the most appropriate therapies for individual patients.

Clinical Data Integration:

Personalized treatment plans consider not only genetic and molecular information but also integrate clinical data, such as tumor stage, patient history, and treatment response. Combining these elements allows for a comprehensive understanding of the patient's disease and facilitates treatment decisions that consider the patient's overall well-being and treatment goals.

Advancements in Personalized Treatment Plans

Targeted Therapies:

Targeted therapies are a key component of personalized treatment plans. These drugs selectively inhibit specific molecular targets involved in tumor growth and progression. By targeting specific vulnerabilities unique to individual patients, targeted therapies can offer more effective treatment options with reduced toxicities compared to traditional chemotherapy. Examples include tyrosine kinase inhibitors, monoclonal antibodies, and immune checkpoint inhibitors.

Immunotherapy:

Immunotherapy has emerged as a transformative approach in cancer treatment. It harnesses the body's immune system to recognize and attack cancer cells. Personalized treatment plans can identify specific biomarkers, such as programmed death-ligand 1 (PD-L1) expression, to predict patient response to immunotherapy drugs. Additionally, the use of tumor-infiltrating lymphocytes (TILs) or chimeric antigen receptor (CAR) T-cell therapy represents promising avenues for personalized immunotherapy.

Liquid Biopsies:

Liquid biopsies offer a non-invasive method for profiling tumors and monitoring treatment response. These tests analyze circulating tumor DNA (ctDNA) or tumor-derived exosomes in blood samples. Liquid biopsies can provide real-time information about tumor genetic alterations, treatment response, and the emergence of resistance mutations. This allows for

## Stages of cancer and chemotherapy

Cancer is a complex disease that progresses through different stages, each characterized by distinct characteristics and implications for treatment. Chemotherapy, a potent tool in cancer therapy, plays a vital role in targeting cancer cells at various stages of the disease. This chapter explores the stages of cancer and how chemotherapy is utilized to combat the disease, providing insights into the multifaceted approach to treatment.

2. Stage 0: Cancer in Situ

At stage 0, cancer is in situ, meaning it is localized and has not spread to nearby tissues or organs. In this early stage, the primary tumor is confined to the site of origin, allowing for more effective treatment options. Surgery is often the preferred approach, as it can remove the tumor entirely. However, chemotherapy may be used as an adjuvant therapy following surgery to eliminate any remaining cancer cells and reduce the risk of recurrence. Adjuvant chemotherapy is particularly beneficial in aggressive cancers with a high risk of metastasis.

3. Stage I and II: Localized Cancer

In stages I and II, cancer is still localized, but there may be some spread to nearby lymph nodes or tissues. Surgery remains the primary treatment, aiming to remove the tumor and affected lymph nodes. However, chemotherapy may be recommended in certain cases. Adjuvant chemotherapy is administered after surgery to eradicate any remaining cancer cells and reduce the risk of recurrence. Neoadjuvant chemotherapy, on the other hand, is given before surgery to shrink the tumor, making it more amenable to surgical removal. Neoadjuvant chemotherapy can also help assess tumor response to treatment and guide further therapy decisions.

4. Stage III: Locally Advanced Cancer

Stage III signifies locally advanced cancer, where the tumor has spread further into surrounding tissues or lymph nodes. At this stage, the cancer may not be amenable to complete surgical removal. Chemotherapy plays a crucial role in the management of stage III cancer, often as part of multimodal treatment. Neoadjuvant chemotherapy is frequently administered to shrink the tumor, making it resectable or reducing the need for extensive surgery. This approach aims to improve surgical outcomes and increase the chances of successful tumor removal. Adjuvant chemotherapy may follow surgery to eliminate any remaining cancer cells and reduce the risk of recurrence.

5. Stage IV: Metastatic Cancer

Stage IV is characterized by the spread of cancer to distant organs or tissues, indicating metastasis. In this advanced stage, the primary goal of treatment shifts from cure to palliation, focusing on symptom management and extending survival. Chemotherapy plays a significant role in managing metastatic cancer. Systemic chemotherapy is administered to target cancer cells throughout the body. The choice of chemotherapy drugs depends on the specific cancer type, patient characteristics, and treatment goals. The aim is to shrink tumors, alleviate symptoms, and prolong life. Targeted therapies, immunotherapy, or combination chemotherapy regimens may be utilized to maximize treatment efficacy and patient outcomes.

Chemotherapy Strategies for Different Stages

Combination Chemotherapy:

Combination chemotherapy involves using multiple chemotherapy drugs with different mechanisms of action. This strategy aims to target cancer cells at various stages of the cell cycle, reduce the risk of drug resistance, and improve treatment efficacy. Combination chemotherapy is often employed in stage III and IV cancers to maximize the chances of response and enhance survival outcomes.

Adjuvant Chemotherapy:

Adjuvant chemotherapy is administered after surgery to eradicate any microscopic cancer cells that may be left behind. It aims to reduce the risk of recurrence and improve long-term survival. Adjuvant chemotherapy is commonly used in stage I, II, and III cancers, depending on the specific characteristics of the tumor and the patient.

Neoadjuvant Chemotherapy:

Neoadjuvant chemotherapy is administered before surgery to

## Determining the correct dosage

Chemotherapy is a powerful treatment modality in the fight against cancer, but determining the correct dosage is crucial to balance effectiveness and minimize side effects. Each patient's response to chemotherapy can vary based on factors such as cancer type, stage, overall health, and individual characteristics. This chapter explores the importance of determining the correct dosage in chemotherapy, highlighting the considerations, methods, and advancements in dosage determination to optimize treatment outcomes.

Considerations in Dosage Determination

Efficacy:

The primary goal of chemotherapy is to eradicate cancer cells or control their growth. Determining the correct dosage is crucial to ensure that sufficient levels of chemotherapy drugs are achieved in the body to effectively target and destroy cancer cells. The dosage should be tailored to the specific cancer type and its response to different drugs.

Tolerance and Toxicity:

Chemotherapy drugs can have significant side effects due to their impact on healthy cells as well. Determining the correct dosage involves finding a balance between delivering a sufficient dose to target cancer cells and minimizing toxicity to healthy tissues. Patient factors such as age, overall health, organ function, and previous treatment history play a crucial role in dosage determination.

Methods of Dosage Determination

Body Surface Area (BSA):

Body surface area-based dosing involves calculating the chemotherapy dosage based on the patient's height and weight. This method takes into account the individual's body size and helps adjust the dosage accordingly. BSA-based dosing is commonly used for drugs with known relationships between body size and drug clearance.

Body Weight:

Body weight-based dosing involves calculating the chemotherapy dosage based on the patient's weight. This method is particularly useful when there is a clear relationship between drug efficacy and body weight. It allows for individualized dosing adjustments based on the patient's weight, ensuring that an appropriate dose is administered.

Maximum Tolerated Dose (MTD):

The maximum tolerated dose refers to the highest dose of a chemotherapy drug that can be given without causing excessive toxicity. Determining the MTD involves conducting clinical trials and carefully monitoring patient responses and side effects. The MTD is then used as a reference point to guide dosage determination in subsequent treatment settings.

Pharmacokinetics:

Pharmacokinetics involves studying how drugs are absorbed, distributed, metabolized, and eliminated from the body. Pharmacokinetic parameters, such as drug clearance and half-life, can help determine the optimal dosage regimen for individual patients. Therapeutic drug monitoring may be employed to measure drug levels in the blood and adjust dosages accordingly.

Advancements in Dosage Determination

Pharmacogenomics:

Pharmacogenomics explores the influence of genetic factors on drug response. Genetic variations can impact how individuals metabolize and respond to chemotherapy drugs. By analyzing specific genetic markers, such as single nucleotide polymorphisms (SNPs), clinicians can tailor dosage and treatment strategies based on an individual's genetic profile. Pharmacogenomic testing is becoming increasingly important in optimizing chemotherapy dosing and reducing the risk of adverse effects.

Therapeutic Drug Monitoring (TDM):

Therapeutic drug monitoring involves measuring drug levels in the blood to ensure that therapeutic concentrations are achieved. By monitoring drug levels, clinicians can optimize dosing regimens, maintain drug efficacy, and minimize toxicity. TDM is particularly relevant for drugs with a narrow therapeutic index, where small changes in dosage can significantly impact treatment outcomes.

Computer Simulations and Modeling:

Computer simulations and modeling techniques are used to predict drug concentrations in the body based on patient-specific factors. These models take into account patient characteristics, drug pharmacokinetics, and tumor response data. By simulating different dosage scenarios, clinicians can optimize treatment regimens and individualize chemotherapy dosing.

Continuous Inf

Chapter Four

# Side Effects and Management

Chemotherapy is a powerful treatment modality in the fight against cancer, but it can come with a range of side effects that affect patients physically, emotionally, and mentally. Understanding and managing these side effects is crucial to ensure the well-being and quality of life of individuals undergoing chemotherapy. This chapter explores the common side effects of chemotherapy and the strategies employed to effectively manage and alleviate them.

Common Side Effects of Chemotherapy

Fatigue:

Fatigue is one of the most prevalent side effects of chemotherapy. It can manifest as physical exhaustion, lack of energy, and decreased motivation. Chemotherapy affects healthy cells along with cancer cells, leading to a general feeling of tiredness. Fatigue can vary in severity and duration, depending on the specific chemotherapy regimen and individual factors.

Nausea and Vomiting:

Nausea and vomiting are common side effects of chemotherapy, particularly with certain drugs. These symptoms can significantly impact a patient's quality of life and nutritional intake. Chemotherapy-induced nausea and vomiting (CINV) can occur immediately after treatment or develop a few days later. Antiemetic medications, such as serotonin receptor antagonists and neurokinin-1 receptor antagonists, are commonly prescribed to prevent and manage CINV.

Hair Loss:

Hair loss, or alopecia, is a distressing side effect of chemotherapy. The drugs can damage hair follicles, leading to partial or complete hair loss on the scalp, eyebrows, eyelashes, and other body areas. Hair loss can have a significant psychological impact on patients, affecting self-esteem and body image. Cold caps, scalp cooling devices, and wig options are available to minimize hair loss or manage its impact.

Decreased Blood Cell Counts:

Chemotherapy can affect the production of blood cells, leading to a decrease in red blood cells, white blood cells, and platelets. This can result in anemia, increased susceptibility to infections, and a higher risk of bleeding. Blood cell counts are closely monitored during chemotherapy, and supportive measures, such as red blood cell transfusions or administration of growth factors, may be employed to manage these effects.

Gastrointestinal Effects:

Chemotherapy drugs can cause a range of gastrointestinal side effects, including diarrhea, constipation, mouth sores, and mucositis. These effects can impact nutritional intake, digestion, and overall comfort. Patients are often advised to follow dietary guidelines, maintain hydration, and use medications to manage these symptoms. Regular oral care and gentle oral hygiene practices are recommended to prevent and manage mouth sores.

Neuropathy:

Chemotherapy-induced peripheral neuropathy (CIPN) is characterized by numbness, tingling, pain, and weakness in the hands and feet. The drugs can damage nerves, leading to these sensory and motor disturbances. CIPN can significantly impact daily activities and quality of life. Medications, physical therapy, and lifestyle modifications are employed to manage neuropathy symptoms.

Management Strategies for Side Effects

Supportive Medications:

Supportive medications, such as antiemetics, pain relievers, and antidiarrheals, are commonly prescribed to manage specific side effects. These medications aim to alleviate symptoms and improve patient comfort. It is important for patients to communicate their symptoms to healthcare providers to receive appropriate supportive care.

Nutritional Support:

Maintaining adequate nutrition is crucial during chemotherapy. A registered dietitian can provide guidance on proper nutrition, diet modifications, and strategies to manage side effects that impact appetite, taste changes, and gastrointestinal function. Ensuring adequate hydration is also important.

Psychological and Emotional Support:

The emotional toll of chemotherapy can be significant, and patients may experience anxiety, depression, and mood changes. Psychological support, counseling, and support groups

## Common side effects

Chemotherapy, a vital component of cancer treatment, can elicit a range of side effects that can significantly impact a patient's well-being. While the benefits of chemotherapy in combating cancer are substantial, managing these side effects is crucial to enhance patient comfort and quality of life. This chapter explores some of the common side effects of chemotherapy and strategies employed to effectively manage and alleviate them.

Fatigue:

Fatigue is one of the most prevalent and distressing side effects experienced by patients undergoing chemotherapy. It is characterized by a persistent feeling of tiredness, lack of energy, and reduced physical and mental stamina. The exact cause of chemotherapy-induced fatigue is not fully understood, but it is thought to result from a combination of factors, including the toxic effects of chemotherapy on healthy cells and the body's response to inflammation.

To manage fatigue, patients are encouraged to prioritize rest and sleep, engage in regular physical activity, and conserve energy by balancing activity and rest periods. Moderate exercise, such as walking or gentle stretching, has been shown to alleviate fatigue and improve overall well-being. Supportive care interventions, such as counseling and relaxation techniques, can also help patients cope with fatigue and enhance their emotional well-being.

Nausea and Vomiting:

Nausea and vomiting are common side effects of chemotherapy and can significantly impact a patient's quality of life. Chemotherapy-induced nausea and vomiting (CINV) can occur immediately after treatment or develop in the days following chemotherapy. The severity and duration of CINV can vary depending on the specific chemotherapy drugs used, individual susceptibility, and the overall treatment regimen.

To manage CINV, patients are often prescribed antiemetic medications, such as serotonin receptor antagonists and neurokinin-1 receptor antagonists. These medications help prevent and control nausea and vomiting by targeting specific receptors in the brain associated with these symptoms. In addition to pharmacological interventions, complementary therapies, such as acupuncture and acupressure, have shown promise in reducing chemotherapy-induced nausea and vomiting.

Hair Loss (Alopecia):

Hair loss, or alopecia, is a distressing side effect of chemotherapy that can have a significant impact on a patient's self-image and emotional well-being. Chemotherapy drugs can damage hair follicles, resulting in partial or complete hair loss on the scalp, eyebrows, eyelashes, and other body areas. The extent and timing of hair loss can vary depending on the specific drugs used and individual factors.

While hair loss cannot be entirely prevented, cooling caps or scalp cooling devices can be used during chemotherapy infusion to reduce blood flow to the scalp and minimize hair loss. Wigs, scarves, and other head coverings can provide cosmetic support and help patients maintain a sense of normalcy during treatment. Support groups, counseling, and individualized support from healthcare professionals can also assist patients in coping with the emotional impact of hair loss.

Changes in Appetite and Weight:

Chemotherapy can affect a patient's appetite and lead to changes in taste preferences, resulting in a loss of appetite or altered food preferences. Additionally, some chemotherapy drugs can cause weight gain or weight loss. These changes in appetite and weight can impact nutritional intake and overall well-being.

Patients are advised to maintain a balanced and nutritious diet during chemotherapy, focusing on consuming small, frequent meals that are easily digestible. Collaborating with a registered dietitian can provide tailored dietary recommendations based on individual needs and preferences. It is important to communicate any significant changes in appetite or weight to healthcare providers for appropriate guidance and support.

Mucositis and Oral Complications:

Mucositis, inflammation and ulceration of the mucous membranes lining the mouth and digestive tract, is a common side effect of chemotherapy. It can result in pain, discomfort,

## Long-term side effects

Chemotherapy is a powerful treatment modality in the fight against cancer, but it can leave a lasting impact on patients even after the completion of treatment. While the immediate side effects of chemotherapy are well-known, long-term side effects can arise months or even years later. Understanding and managing these long-term side effects is crucial to ensure the ongoing well-being and quality of life of cancer survivors. This chapter explores some of the common long-term side effects of chemotherapy and strategies employed to address and mitigate their impact.

Cognitive Changes (Chemobrain):

Cognitive changes, commonly referred to as "chemobrain," are often reported by cancer survivors who have undergone chemotherapy. Chemobrain encompasses a range of cognitive symptoms, including memory problems, difficulty concentrating, and decreased mental clarity. These symptoms can persist for months or even years after the completion of treatment.

The exact causes of chemobrain are not fully understood but may involve chemotherapy's impact on the central nervous system, inflammation, hormonal changes, and psychological factors. Strategies to manage chemobrain include cognitive rehabilitation programs, memory exercises, stress reduction techniques, and lifestyle modifications such as regular physical exercise and a healthy diet. Supportive care interventions, such as counseling and support groups, can also help patients cope with the emotional and psychological aspects of chemobrain.

Cardiovascular Complications:

Certain chemotherapy drugs, particularly those from the anthracycline class, can have long-term effects on the cardiovascular system. These drugs can cause damage to the heart muscle, leading to a condition called cardiomyopathy, which can result in heart failure. Radiation therapy to the chest area can also contribute to cardiovascular complications.

To monitor and manage cardiovascular risks, cancer survivors may undergo regular cardiac assessments, such as echocardiograms or cardiac stress tests, to evaluate heart function. Lifestyle modifications, including a heart-healthy diet, regular exercise, and avoiding tobacco use, are crucial for long-term cardiovascular health. Medications, such as ACE inhibitors or beta-blockers, may be prescribed to manage cardiac complications.

Secondary Cancers:

While chemotherapy is aimed at targeting cancer cells, certain chemotherapy drugs can increase the risk of developing secondary cancers later in life. This risk is influenced by factors such as the specific drugs used, cumulative doses, and individual susceptibility. Common secondary cancers associated with chemotherapy include leukemia, myelodysplastic syndromes, and solid tumors.

Long-term surveillance is essential for early detection and management of secondary cancers. Cancer survivors are advised to undergo regular screenings and follow-up appointments as recommended by their healthcare providers. Lifestyle factors, such as maintaining a healthy weight, avoiding tobacco use, and reducing exposure to environmental carcinogens, can also help minimize the risk of developing secondary cancers.

Infertility and Sexual Dysfunction:

Chemotherapy can have significant impacts on reproductive function, leading to temporary or permanent infertility in both men and women. In women, chemotherapy drugs can damage the ovaries and disrupt hormonal balance, potentially leading to menstrual irregularities, early menopause, or infertility. In men, chemotherapy can affect sperm production and quality.

Patients of reproductive age who are planning to undergo chemotherapy may consider fertility preservation options, such as egg or sperm freezing, prior to treatment. For those experiencing infertility or sexual dysfunction as a result of chemotherapy, assisted reproductive techniques, hormone replacement therapy, or counseling may be helpful in addressing these concerns.

Psychological and Emotional Impact:

The psychological and emotional impact of chemotherapy can extend beyond the treatment period, affecting the long-term well-being of cancer survivors. Many individuals experience anxiety, depression, fear of recurrence, post-traumatic stress symptoms, and changes in body image after chemotherapy.

Psychosocial support, counseling, and support groups play a crucial role in addressing the psychological and emotional challenges

## Tips for managing side effects

Chemotherapy is a powerful treatment modality in the fight against cancer, but it can be accompanied by a range of side effects that can impact a patient's well-being. Managing these side effects effectively is crucial to enhance patient comfort and quality of life during treatment. This chapter provides practical tips and strategies for patients undergoing chemotherapy to help them navigate and minimize the impact of common side effects.

Communicate with Your Healthcare Team:

Open and honest communication with your healthcare team is vital throughout your chemotherapy journey. They are equipped to provide guidance, support, and interventions to help manage side effects. Discuss any symptoms or concerns you experience, even if you think they may be minor. Your healthcare team can offer tailored recommendations and adjustments to your treatment plan to address specific side effects.

Follow a Healthy Diet:

Maintaining proper nutrition is crucial during chemotherapy. Eat a balanced diet that includes a variety of fruits, vegetables, whole grains, lean proteins, and healthy fats. Consider working with a registered dietitian who specializes in oncology to develop a personalized nutrition plan. They can provide guidance on managing specific side effects, such as nausea, taste changes, or mouth sores, and suggest dietary modifications to support your overall well-being.

Stay Hydrated:

Chemotherapy and its side effects can increase the risk of dehydration. Drink plenty of fluids throughout the day, aiming for at least eight glasses of water. If you have difficulty drinking large amounts of fluids at once, try sipping fluids throughout the day or using a straw. Monitor your urine color and aim for a pale yellow color as an indicator of adequate hydration.

Engage in Regular Exercise:

Physical activity can help combat fatigue, improve mood, and enhance overall well-being during chemotherapy. Engage in regular exercise, even if it's low intensity or light activities such as walking, stretching, or gentle yoga. Consult with your healthcare team before starting an exercise regimen to ensure it is safe and appropriate for your specific situation.

Prioritize Rest and Sleep:

Fatigue is a common side effect of chemotherapy, and getting sufficient rest and quality sleep is essential. Listen to your body and prioritize rest when needed. Establish a regular sleep routine, ensuring a quiet and comfortable sleeping environment. If you experience difficulties sleeping, consider relaxation techniques, such as deep breathing exercises or guided imagery, to promote relaxation and improve sleep quality.

Utilize Supportive Care Measures:

Supportive care measures can help alleviate and manage specific side effects. For example, if you experience chemotherapy-induced nausea and vomiting, follow the prescribed antiemetic regimen as directed by your healthcare team. If you develop mouth sores, practice good oral hygiene and use recommended mouth rinses or gels. For hair loss, explore options such as wigs, scarves, or hats to maintain a sense of normalcy and boost confidence.

Seek Emotional Support:

Emotional well-being is vital during chemotherapy. Reach out to friends, family, and support groups for emotional support. Consider joining support groups or seeking counseling services specifically tailored for cancer patients. These resources can provide a safe space to share experiences, express emotions, and receive guidance in managing the emotional challenges of chemotherapy.

Communicate with Others:

Inform your family, friends, and coworkers about your chemotherapy journey. Educate them about common side effects and potential changes in your energy levels or physical appearance. By fostering understanding and open communication, you create a supportive environment that can alleviate stress and enhance your emotional well-being.

Practice Self-Care:

Prioritize self-care activities that bring you joy and relaxation. Engage in activities such as reading, listening to music, practicing mindfulness, taking warm baths, or pursuing hobbies. Self-care activities can help reduce stress, improve mood, and

Chapter Five

# Chemotherapy and the Immune System

Chemotherapy, a cornerstone of cancer treatment, plays a critical role in targeting and destroying cancer cells. However, its impact extends beyond the tumor, affecting various components of the immune system. The immune system, responsible for defending the body against pathogens and abnormal cells, can be both a beneficiary and a victim of chemotherapy. This chapter explores the dynamic relationship between chemotherapy and the immune system, shedding light on the effects of chemotherapy on immune function and strategies employed to optimize immune health during treatment.

Effects of Chemotherapy on the Immune System

Suppression of Immune Cells:

Chemotherapy drugs can have suppressive effects on various immune cells, including white blood cells (leukocytes), which are integral to immune defense. Chemotherapy may lead to a decrease in the production of immune cells in the bone marrow, impair their function, or induce their destruction. This can result in a weakened immune response and increased susceptibility to infections.

Impact on Lymphocytes:

Lymphocytes, a type of white blood cell, play a crucial role in immune defense. Chemotherapy can decrease the number of lymphocytes, particularly T cells and B cells, impairing their ability to recognize and eliminate abnormal cells. This reduction in lymphocyte levels can lead to a compromised immune response, making the body more vulnerable to infections and other illnesses.

Disruption of the Bone Marrow:

Chemotherapy drugs can damage the bone marrow, the site of blood cell production. This damage may affect the production of white blood cells, red blood cells, and platelets. Reductions in white blood cell counts, specifically neutrophils, can result in neutropenia, a condition characterized by a decreased ability to fight infections.

Strategies to Optimize Immune Health during Chemotherapy

Supportive Care:

Supportive care measures aim to mitigate the impact of chemotherapy on the immune system and reduce the risk of infections. These measures may include the administration of growth factors, such as granulocyte colony-stimulating factor (G-CSF), to stimulate the production of white blood cells. Prophylactic antibiotics may be prescribed to prevent or treat infections, particularly in individuals with low white blood cell counts.

Vaccinations:

Vaccinations can help enhance immune protection during chemotherapy. It is recommended that cancer patients receive appropriate vaccinations prior to starting treatment, as their immune response may be compromised during therapy. Vaccinations for influenza, pneumonia, and other preventable infections can help reduce the risk of complications and maintain immune health.

Infection Prevention:

Practicing good hygiene and infection prevention measures is crucial for individuals undergoing chemotherapy. This includes regular handwashing, avoiding close contact with individuals who are sick, and maintaining a clean environment. It is advisable to follow specific precautions recommended by healthcare providers to reduce the risk of infection, such as wearing masks or avoiding crowded places.

Nutritional Support:

Maintaining proper nutrition is essential for optimal immune function. A balanced diet that includes a variety of fruits, vegetables, whole grains, lean proteins, and healthy fats provides essential nutrients and antioxidants to support immune health. Consultation with a registered dietitian who specializes in oncology can help develop a personalized nutrition plan to meet individual needs during chemotherapy.

Physical Activity:

Engaging in regular physical activity, as allowed by healthcare providers, can help support immune function during chemotherapy. Exercise has been shown to have immune-enhancing effects and improve overall well-being. However, it is important to consult with healthcare professionals before starting an exercise regimen, as individual limitations and considerations may apply.

Stress Reduction:

Chronic stress can negatively impact immune function. Managing stress through relaxation techniques, mindfulness practices, and stress reduction strategies can support immune health during chemotherapy. Patients may explore activities such

## Effects on white blood cells

Chemotherapy, a potent treatment for cancer, exerts a wide range of effects on the body's cells, including white blood cells. White blood cells, also known as leukocytes, play a vital role in the immune response, defending the body against infections and abnormal cells. However, chemotherapy can disrupt the delicate balance of white blood cell production and function, leading to potential consequences for the immune system. This chapter delves into the impact of chemotherapy on white blood cells, shedding light on the effects and strategies employed to manage these changes during treatment.

Decreased White Blood Cell Counts:

Chemotherapy can cause a decrease in white blood cell counts, a condition known as leukopenia. This reduction primarily affects neutrophils, a type of white blood cell crucial for fighting bacterial infections. Neutropenia, characterized by low neutrophil counts, increases the risk of infections and can result in prolonged recovery periods from infections when they do occur. The severity and duration of neutropenia depend on the specific chemotherapy drugs, dosages, and treatment regimens employed.

Impaired Immune Function:

Chemotherapy can impair the overall function of white blood cells, compromising the immune response. T cells and B cells, two essential types of lymphocytes involved in adaptive immunity, may be affected. Chemotherapy drugs can disrupt the production, maturation, and activation of these cells, leading to a weakened immune defense against infections and abnormal cells.

Increased Susceptibility to Infections:

A decrease in white blood cell counts, particularly neutrophils, renders individuals undergoing chemotherapy more susceptible to infections. The immune system's ability to recognize, respond to, and eliminate pathogens is compromised. Even minor infections, such as urinary tract infections or respiratory infections, can pose significant risks and require prompt medical attention.

Strategies to Manage White Blood Cell Changes during Chemotherapy

Supportive Medications:

Supportive medications can help manage white blood cell changes during chemotherapy. Growth factors, such as granulocyte colony-stimulating factor (G-CSF), can stimulate the production of white blood cells, particularly neutrophils. G-CSF is commonly used in cases of high-risk neutropenia or when chemotherapy regimens are associated with a higher incidence of neutropenia. These medications can reduce the duration and severity of neutropenia, thereby minimizing the risk of infections.

Prophylactic Antibiotics:

Prophylactic antibiotics may be prescribed to prevent infections in individuals with chemotherapy-induced neutropenia. Antibiotics are administered as a preventive measure to reduce the risk of bacterial infections. They are typically prescribed to patients with severe neutropenia, a history of recurrent infections, or specific risk factors for infections. Prophylactic antibiotics can help safeguard individuals during periods of heightened vulnerability to bacterial pathogens.

Neutropenic Precautions:

Individuals with chemotherapy-induced neutropenia are advised to follow neutropenic precautions to minimize the risk of infections. These precautions include maintaining good hygiene practices, such as frequent handwashing, avoiding close contact with individuals who are sick, and practicing good oral hygiene. It is advisable to adhere to specific guidelines provided by healthcare providers to reduce the risk of infection and maintain overall well-being.

Timing of Chemotherapy Administration:

The timing of chemotherapy administration can be adjusted to manage white blood cell changes. Dose delays or adjustments may be considered if there is significant neutropenia or the recovery of white blood cell counts is slower than expected. This allows for the optimization of chemotherapy regimens while minimizing the risk of complications associated with low white blood cell counts.

Monitoring White Blood Cell Counts:

Regular monitoring of white blood cell counts is essential during chemotherapy. Blood tests, such as complete blood counts (

## Neutropenia and infection risk

Chemotherapy, a potent treatment for cancer, can have significant impacts on the body's immune system, particularly on white blood cells. Neutropenia, a condition characterized by low levels of neutrophils, a type of white blood cell crucial for fighting bacterial infections, is a common consequence of chemotherapy. Neutropenia increases the risk of infections and poses challenges for individuals undergoing treatment. This chapter explores the relationship between neutropenia and infection risk, shedding light on the implications and strategies employed to manage this vulnerability during chemotherapy.

Understanding Neutropenia:

Neutropenia refers to a decrease in the absolute neutrophil count (ANC), which measures the number of neutrophils in the blood. Neutrophils are the body's first line of defense against bacterial infections. Chemotherapy can suppress the bone marrow, where white blood cells are produced, resulting in reduced neutrophil counts. The severity and duration of neutropenia can vary depending on the specific chemotherapy drugs, dosages, and treatment regimens used.

Infection Risk during Neutropenia:

Neutropenia significantly increases the risk of infections, particularly bacterial infections. With low neutrophil counts, the body's ability to recognize, respond to, and eliminate bacteria is compromised. Common sources of infection during neutropenia include the respiratory tract, urinary tract, skin, and gastrointestinal tract. Even minor infections can rapidly escalate and lead to severe complications if not promptly diagnosed and treated.

Strategies to Manage Infection Risk during Neutropenia:

Neutropenic Precautions:

Individuals with neutropenia are advised to follow neutropenic precautions to minimize the risk of infections. These precautions include practicing good hand hygiene, such as frequent handwashing with soap and water or alcohol-based hand sanitizers. It is important to avoid close contact with individuals who have infections, and wearing masks may be recommended in certain situations. Following these precautions can help reduce exposure to potential pathogens.

Environmental Precautions:

Maintaining a clean and hygienic environment is crucial during neutropenia. Regular cleaning of frequently touched surfaces, such as doorknobs, light switches, and countertops, with disinfectants can help minimize the presence of harmful bacteria. Avoiding overcrowded places and large gatherings can also reduce the risk of exposure to infectious agents.

Prompt Recognition and Treatment of Infections:

Vigilance in recognizing the signs and symptoms of infection is essential during neutropenia. Even subtle changes, such as fever, cough, urinary symptoms, or skin abnormalities, should be promptly reported to healthcare providers. Early detection allows for timely initiation of appropriate antibiotic therapy and reduces the risk of complications.

Prophylactic Antibiotics:

Prophylactic antibiotics may be prescribed to prevent infections in individuals with a high risk of developing neutropenic infections. These antibiotics are administered preemptively, often in cases of severe neutropenia or specific risk factors for infections. Prophylactic antibiotics can help reduce the incidence of infections and their associated complications.

Growth Factors:

Growth factors, such as granulocyte colony-stimulating factor (G-CSF), are commonly used to stimulate the production and maturation of neutrophils. These medications can help reduce the duration and severity of neutropenia, thereby lowering the risk of infections. G-CSF is often administered in certain chemotherapy regimens associated with a higher incidence of neutropenia or in cases where the risk of infection is significant.

Timing of Chemotherapy Administration:

The timing of chemotherapy administration can be adjusted to minimize the duration and impact of neutropenia. Dose delays or adjustments may be considered if there is significant neutropenia or

## Boosting immune health during treatment

Chemotherapy, a powerful tool in cancer treatment, can have a significant impact on the immune system. During chemotherapy, it is crucial to support and boost immune health to optimize the body's ability to fight infections and maintain overall well-being. This chapter explores strategies and lifestyle modifications that can help boost immune health during chemotherapy, empowering individuals to navigate their treatment journey with resilience.

Nutrient-Rich Diet:

Eating a nutrient-rich diet is essential for supporting immune health during chemotherapy. Include a variety of fruits, vegetables, whole grains, lean proteins, and healthy fats in your meals. These foods provide essential vitamins, minerals, and antioxidants that support immune function. Vitamin C, found in citrus fruits, strawberries, and bell peppers, is particularly known for its immune-boosting properties. Zinc, found in nuts, seeds, and legumes, is also important for immune health.

Hydration:

Staying hydrated is crucial for optimal immune function. Drinking adequate water and fluids helps transport nutrients throughout the body and supports the elimination of waste products. Aim to drink at least eight glasses of water per day, and increase fluid intake if experiencing diarrhea or vomiting. If plain water is unappealing, try infused water with fruits or herbal teas to make hydration more enjoyable.

Regular Exercise:

Engaging in regular exercise can have a positive impact on immune health during chemotherapy. Exercise helps improve circulation, reduce inflammation, and enhance the production and activity of immune cells. Incorporate moderate-intensity exercises, such as walking, swimming, or cycling, into your routine, aiming for at least 30 minutes of activity most days of the week. Consult with your healthcare team before starting an exercise program to ensure it is safe and appropriate for your condition.

Adequate Sleep:

Quality sleep plays a vital role in immune health. During sleep, the body repairs and rejuvenates itself, supporting immune function. Aim for seven to eight hours of uninterrupted sleep each night. Establish a regular sleep routine by going to bed and waking up at consistent times. Create a sleep-friendly environment by keeping your bedroom cool, dark, and quiet. If sleep disturbances persist, discuss them with your healthcare team for appropriate management strategies.

Stress Management:

Chronic stress can weaken the immune system. Finding effective ways to manage stress is essential during chemotherapy. Explore stress reduction techniques such as deep breathing exercises, meditation, mindfulness, and relaxation practices. Engaging in activities that bring you joy, such as hobbies, listening to music, or spending time in nature, can also help alleviate stress and promote emotional well-being.

Supportive Herbs and Supplements:

Certain herbs and supplements may support immune health during chemotherapy. However, it is essential to consult with your healthcare team before starting any new supplements to ensure they do not interfere with your treatment or have adverse effects. Some commonly used supplements for immune support include vitamin D, probiotics, medicinal mushrooms (such as reishi and shiitake), and herbal teas like echinacea or green tea. These supplements should be used judiciously and under professional guidance.

Mindful Hand Hygiene:

Maintaining proper hand hygiene is crucial during chemotherapy to reduce the risk of infections. Wash your hands regularly with soap and water for at least 20 seconds, especially before eating, after using the bathroom, or touching potentially contaminated surfaces. If soap and water are not readily available, use alcohol-based hand sanitizers. Avoid touching your face, nose, or mouth to minimize the entry of pathogens into your body.

Avoidance of Potential Infections:

During chemotherapy, it is important to minimize exposure to potential infections. Avoid close contact with individuals who are sick or have contagious illnesses. Consider wearing a mask in crowded places or when

Chapter Six

# Nutrition During Chemotherapy

Chemotherapy, a potent treatment for cancer, can take a toll on the body, affecting appetite, digestion, and nutrient absorption. Proper nutrition during chemotherapy is essential to provide the body with the fuel and building blocks it needs to withstand the treatment's demands and support overall well-being. This chapter explores the importance of nutrition during chemotherapy, provides insights into common challenges, and offers practical tips to optimize nutritional intake during treatment.

Maintaining Adequate Caloric Intake:

Chemotherapy can lead to a decrease in appetite, changes in taste preferences, and gastrointestinal side effects, which can affect the ability to consume adequate calories. However, it is crucial to provide the body with enough energy to support healing and prevent malnutrition. Here are some strategies to consider:

Frequent, Small Meals:

Instead of three large meals, try consuming five to six smaller meals throughout the day. This approach can help overcome a reduced appetite and make eating more manageable.

Calorie-Dense Foods:

Incorporate calorie-dense foods into your meals and snacks. Nut butters, avocados, nuts, seeds, dried fruits, and full-fat dairy products can add extra calories without requiring larger portions.

Nutritional Supplements:

Consider nutritional supplements, such as meal replacement shakes or high-calorie drinks, to bridge any gaps in caloric intake. These can be particularly helpful when appetite is low or when managing side effects that impact eating.

Meeting Nutrient Needs:

Chemotherapy can impact nutrient absorption and increase nutrient requirements. Ensuring adequate intake of key nutrients is crucial during treatment. Here are some nutrient-specific considerations:

Protein:

Protein is essential for tissue repair and immune function. Aim to include protein-rich foods in each meal and snack, such as lean meats, poultry, fish, dairy products, legumes, and tofu. If digestion or taste changes make it challenging to consume protein-rich foods, consider protein supplements or shakes recommended by your healthcare team.

Vitamins and Minerals:

Chemotherapy can deplete certain vitamins and minerals. Focus on consuming a varied and colorful diet that includes fruits, vegetables, whole grains, and lean proteins to obtain a wide range of essential nutrients. Your healthcare team may recommend specific supplements based on your individual needs.

Hydration:

Maintaining proper hydration is essential during chemotherapy. Some chemotherapy drugs can cause fluid loss, and side effects like vomiting or diarrhea can further deplete fluids. Drink plenty of water throughout the day and include hydrating foods like soups, broths, fruits, and vegetables. If hydration is challenging, consult your healthcare team for additional guidance.

Managing Gastrointestinal Side Effects:

Chemotherapy can cause various gastrointestinal side effects, including nausea, vomiting, diarrhea, constipation, and mouth sores. These side effects can make it difficult to maintain proper nutrition. Consider the following strategies:

Nausea and Vomiting:

Eat smaller, more frequent meals and choose bland, easy-to-digest foods. Avoid strong-smelling or greasy foods. Ginger, peppermint, and other herbal remedies may help alleviate nausea. Consult with your healthcare team regarding anti-nausea medications, if necessary.

Diarrhea:

Increase fiber intake gradually to help regulate bowel movements. Opt for soluble fiber found in oats, cooked vegetables, and fruits. Avoid high-fiber or greasy foods that can exacerbate diarrhea. Stay hydrated and consult with your healthcare team for appropriate management strategies.

Constipation:

Increase fiber intake by consuming whole grains, fruits, vegetables, and legumes. Stay hydrated and engage in regular physical activity. If necessary, your healthcare team may recommend stool softeners or other medications to alleviate constipation.

Mouth Sores:

Choose soft, moist,

## Dietary recommendations

Chemotherapy, a powerful treatment for cancer, can pose unique challenges when it comes to maintaining proper nutrition. The side effects of chemotherapy can affect appetite, taste preferences, and digestion, making it crucial to provide the body with the right nutrients to support healing and overall well-being. This chapter explores important dietary recommendations during chemotherapy, offering practical tips to optimize nutrition and enhance the body's ability to tolerate treatment.

Emphasize a Plant-Based Diet:

A plant-based diet rich in fruits, vegetables, whole grains, and legumes provides a wide range of essential nutrients, including vitamins, minerals, antioxidants, and dietary fiber. These foods promote overall health, support immune function, and provide necessary energy during chemotherapy. Aim to fill at least half of your plate with colorful fruits and vegetables, incorporate whole grains, and include plant-based protein sources like beans, lentils, and tofu.

Choose Lean Protein Sources:

Protein is essential for tissue repair and immune function. Opt for lean protein sources such as skinless poultry, fish, eggs, low-fat dairy products, legumes, and tofu. These foods provide high-quality protein without excessive amounts of saturated fats. If animal proteins are not well-tolerated, consider plant-based alternatives like lentils, chickpeas, or quinoa.

Stay Hydrated:

Proper hydration is crucial during chemotherapy to support overall health and counteract potential side effects. Drink plenty of water throughout the day, aiming for at least eight cups. Include hydrating foods such as fruits, vegetables, soups, and broths. If nausea or vomiting is a concern, try consuming small sips of water or sucking on ice chips throughout the day. Consult with your healthcare team if fluid intake needs additional attention.

Opt for Healthy Fats:

Include healthy fats in your diet to provide essential fatty acids and promote satiety. Choose sources such as avocados, nuts, seeds, olive oil, and fatty fish like salmon or mackerel. These foods offer valuable nutrients and can enhance the absorption of fat-soluble vitamins. However, moderation is key, as fats are calorie-dense, and excessive intake can contribute to weight gain.

Prioritize Whole Foods:

During chemotherapy, it is essential to focus on whole foods rather than relying heavily on processed or convenience foods. Whole foods are minimally processed, providing a higher concentration of nutrients and reducing the intake of additives, preservatives, and artificial ingredients. Prepare meals using fresh ingredients whenever possible, and limit the consumption of pre-packaged meals, sugary snacks, and beverages.

Manage Nausea and Digestive Issues:

Nausea, vomiting, and digestive issues are common side effects of chemotherapy that can impact nutritional intake. Consider the following strategies:

Eat small, frequent meals throughout the day to prevent feelings of fullness.

Choose foods that are easy to digest, such as bland, lightly seasoned options.

Opt for cooler or room temperature foods if hot or strong-smelling foods worsen symptoms.

Try ginger, peppermint, or chamomile tea, which may help alleviate nausea.

Discuss with your healthcare team about anti-nausea medications that can help manage symptoms.

Pay Attention to Food Safety:

During chemotherapy, the immune system may be compromised, increasing the susceptibility to foodborne illnesses. Practice proper food safety to reduce the risk of infections:

Wash hands thoroughly before handling food and ensure kitchen surfaces and utensils are clean.

Avoid consuming raw or undercooked foods, including eggs, seafood, and meats.

Store perishable foods at appropriate temperatures and discard any expired or spoiled items.

## Managing appetite and weight changes

Chemotherapy, a potent treatment for cancer, can often lead to changes in appetite and weight. Some individuals may experience a loss of appetite, while others may struggle with weight gain. These changes can impact overall nutritional health and well-being, making it crucial to address them effectively. This chapter explores strategies to manage appetite and weight changes during chemotherapy, providing practical tips to support optimal nutrition and overall quality of life.

Communicate with your healthcare team:

Open and honest communication with your healthcare team is essential when it comes to managing appetite and weight changes. They can provide guidance tailored to your specific situation and help address any concerns or challenges you may be experiencing. They may recommend dietary modifications or suggest medications to stimulate appetite or manage weight changes. Regular check-ins with your healthcare team can ensure you are receiving the necessary support throughout your treatment.

Eat Small, Frequent Meals:

If you have a decreased appetite or difficulty eating larger meals, consider consuming smaller, more frequent meals throughout the day. This approach can help you meet your nutritional needs while avoiding overwhelming feelings of fullness. Focus on nutrient-dense foods, such as fruits, vegetables, lean proteins, and whole grains, to maximize the nutritional content of each meal.

Opt for Nutrient-Dense Foods:

During chemotherapy, it is important to prioritize nutrient-dense foods that provide essential vitamins, minerals, and antioxidants. Choose foods such as lean proteins, whole grains, fruits, vegetables, and healthy fats. These foods offer valuable nutrients while minimizing excessive calorie intake. Including a variety of colors and textures in your meals can make them more appealing and enjoyable.

Experiment with Flavors and Textures:

Changes in taste perception during chemotherapy can influence food preferences. Some individuals may experience a metallic taste or find certain foods unappealing. Experiment with different flavors and textures to find what works best for you. Adding herbs, spices, and citrus flavors to meals can enhance taste. Trying different cooking methods, such as grilling, roasting, or steaming, can also impact the texture and flavor of foods.

Stay Hydrated:

Proper hydration is essential for overall health, particularly during chemotherapy. However, some individuals may find it challenging to drink enough fluids due to changes in taste or nausea. Experiment with different fluids, such as flavored water, herbal teas, or diluted fruit juices, to make hydration more appealing. Sipping fluids throughout the day or using a straw can also help increase fluid intake.

Manage Weight Changes:

Weight gain or loss during chemotherapy can have significant impacts on overall well-being. If you experience weight gain, focus on portion control, and choose nutrient-dense, low-calorie foods. Incorporate regular physical activity into your routine, with guidance from your healthcare team, to support weight management. If weight loss is a concern, consider adding calorie-dense foods to your meals, such as avocados, nuts, nut butter, and healthy oils.

Seek Support from a Registered Dietitian:

A registered dietitian specializing in oncology can provide personalized guidance and support in managing appetite and weight changes. They can assess your nutritional needs, develop customized meal plans, and address any specific concerns you may have. They can also provide education on portion control, meal timing, and strategies to improve nutritional intake.

Consider Nutritional Supplements:

In some cases, nutritional supplements may be recommended to ensure adequate nutrient intake during chemotherapy. These supplements can provide additional calories, protein, vitamins, and minerals. Talk to your healthcare team or registered dietitian about the appropriateness of nutritional supplements for your individual needs.

Practice Mindful Eating:

Mindful eating involves being present and attentive while consuming food. Take the time to savor each bite, pay attention

## Hydration and chemotherapy

Hydration plays a crucial role in supporting overall health, especially during chemotherapy. Chemotherapy treatments can cause various side effects that affect hydration status, including nausea, vomiting, diarrhea, and increased fluid loss. Adequate hydration is vital for maintaining proper bodily functions, supporting treatment effectiveness, and minimizing treatment-related complications. This chapter explores the importance of hydration during chemotherapy and provides practical strategies for achieving optimal hydration.

The Significance of Hydration during Chemotherapy:

Chemotherapy drugs can have several effects on the body, including increased fluid loss through urine, vomiting, diarrhea, and sweating. These factors can contribute to dehydration if not properly managed. Dehydration can lead to fatigue, dizziness, constipation, kidney problems, and other complications that can negatively impact the effectiveness of chemotherapy and overall well-being. Therefore, maintaining proper hydration is essential to support the body's functions during treatment.

Guidelines for Hydration:

The general recommendation for daily fluid intake is about 8 cups (64 ounces) for adults. However, during chemotherapy, additional fluid intake may be necessary to compensate for fluid losses and support the body's needs. It is advisable to consult with your healthcare team to determine your specific fluid requirements based on factors such as body weight, treatment regimen, and overall health.

Choosing the Right Fluids:

While water is the primary source of hydration, there are other fluid options that can contribute to overall hydration during chemotherapy. Herbal teas, diluted fruit juices, broths, and electrolyte-rich beverages can be beneficial, particularly if nausea or taste changes make plain water less appealing. It is important to limit or avoid caffeinated and sugary beverages as they can contribute to dehydration.

Sip Fluids Regularly:

Rather than consuming large amounts of fluids at once, it is beneficial to sip fluids regularly throughout the day. This approach helps maintain a consistent level of hydration and reduces the likelihood of overwhelming the stomach, which may be sensitive during chemotherapy. Setting reminders or using water bottles with measured markings can help you track your fluid intake and ensure regular sipping.

Addressing Nausea and Vomiting:

Nausea and vomiting are common side effects of chemotherapy that can impact fluid intake. If you experience these symptoms, it is essential to address them promptly to maintain hydration. Talk to your healthcare team about medications or natural remedies that can help manage nausea and vomiting. They may also suggest specific fluids or strategies to ease these symptoms and promote hydration.

Managing Diarrhea:

Chemotherapy can sometimes cause diarrhea, which can lead to fluid loss and dehydration. If you experience diarrhea, it is important to increase your fluid intake to compensate for the extra fluid loss. Your healthcare team may recommend oral rehydration solutions or electrolyte-rich beverages to help restore the balance of fluids and electrolytes in your body.

Enhancing Hydration with Foods:

In addition to fluids, certain foods can contribute to hydration. Consuming water-rich fruits and vegetables, such as watermelon, cucumbers, oranges, and strawberries, can provide both hydration and essential nutrients. Soups, smoothies, and popsicles made with hydrating ingredients can also be refreshing options.

Overcoming Taste Changes:

Chemotherapy can sometimes alter the taste buds, making water and other fluids taste unpleasant. Experiment with different temperatures, flavors, and textures to find fluids that are more palatable. Adding a squeeze of lemon, cucumber slices, or fresh herbs can enhance the taste and make fluids more enjoyable.

Be Mindful of Fluid Restrictions:

In some cases, certain chemotherapy drugs or treatment plans may require fluid restrictions. It is important to follow the guidelines provided by your healthcare team in such situations. They will consider your specific medical condition and treatment requirements to ensure

Chapter Seven

# Emotional Well-being and Coping Strategies

Chemotherapy, a powerful treatment for cancer, can have profound effects not only on the physical body but also on emotional well-being. The diagnosis, treatment process, side effects, and overall journey can evoke a range of emotions, including fear, anxiety, sadness, and stress. Taking care of your emotional well-being is essential during chemotherapy to maintain overall quality of life and support the healing process. This chapter explores the importance of emotional well-being during chemotherapy and provides practical coping strategies to nurture mental health and resilience.

Acknowledge Your Emotions:

It is normal to experience a wide range of emotions during chemotherapy. Acknowledge and accept your feelings, whether they are positive or negative. Give yourself permission to feel and express your emotions, as suppressing them can lead to increased stress and emotional distress. Consider journaling, talking to a trusted friend or family member, or seeking professional counseling or support groups to process and navigate your emotions.

Seek Support:

Building a strong support system is crucial during chemotherapy. Reach out to loved ones, friends, or support groups who can provide a listening ear, understanding, and encouragement. Consider joining cancer support groups, where you can connect with others going through similar experiences. Additionally, professional counseling or therapy can offer a safe space to explore your emotions, gain coping strategies, and develop resilience.

Practice Self-Care:

Self-care is essential for nurturing emotional well-being during chemotherapy. Set aside time for activities that bring you joy and relaxation. Engage in hobbies, practice mindfulness or meditation, take walks in nature, listen to soothing music, or indulge in activities that promote self-expression, such as art or writing. Prioritize self-care as a vital component of your treatment plan.

Communicate with Your Healthcare Team:

Maintaining open and honest communication with your healthcare team is crucial for addressing emotional concerns. Share your feelings and concerns with them, as they can provide guidance, resources, and referrals to supportive services. They may recommend mental health professionals, support groups, or additional interventions to support your emotional well-being.

Educate Yourself:

Understanding the chemotherapy process and potential side effects can help alleviate anxiety and fear. Educate yourself about the treatment, its purpose, and common side effects. Consult reliable sources, such as reputable medical websites or educational materials provided by your healthcare team. Having accurate information can empower you to make informed decisions and feel more in control of your journey.

Practice Stress Reduction Techniques:

Chemotherapy can induce stress, and finding effective stress reduction techniques can significantly impact emotional well-being. Explore stress management techniques that resonate with you, such as deep breathing exercises, progressive muscle relaxation, guided imagery, or yoga. Engaging in these practices regularly can help reduce stress, promote relaxation, and enhance overall well-being.

Maintain a Routine:

Maintaining a daily routine can provide structure and stability during chemotherapy. Establishing a sense of normalcy and predictability can contribute to a more stable emotional state. Plan your days with a balance of rest, activities, self-care, and social interactions. However, be flexible and adapt your routine as needed to accommodate treatment schedules and any physical limitations.

Practice Positive Self-Talk:

Pay attention to your inner dialogue and consciously replace negative thoughts with positive affirmations. Positive self-talk can help build resilience, boost self-esteem, and foster a more optimistic mindset. Remind yourself of your strengths, celebrate small victories, and focus on the progress you are making. Surround yourself with positive influences and supportive individuals who uplift and encourage you.

Engage in Physical Activity:

Regular physical activity can have a positive impact on emotional well-being during chemotherapy. Engaging in moderate exercise, with guidance from your healthcare team, can improve

## Psychological effects of chemotherapy

Chemotherapy, a vital treatment for cancer, not only targets cancer cells but can also have profound psychological effects on individuals undergoing the treatment. The diagnosis, treatment process, side effects, and uncertainty surrounding the outcome can trigger a range of emotional responses, including anxiety, depression, fear, and stress. Understanding and addressing the psychological effects of chemotherapy are essential for comprehensive care and well-being. This chapter explores the psychological effects of chemotherapy and offers insights into managing the emotional journey with resilience and support.

Anxiety and Fear:

Anxiety and fear are common emotional responses to chemotherapy. The uncertainty surrounding the treatment outcomes, potential side effects, and impact on daily life can generate apprehension. Techniques such as deep breathing, mindfulness, and relaxation exercises can help manage anxiety. Connecting with support networks, participating in support groups, and seeking professional counseling can provide valuable tools for coping with anxiety and fear.

Depression and Mood Changes:

Chemotherapy can also contribute to depression and mood changes. The physical impact of treatment, side effects, and the disruption of daily routines can lead to feelings of sadness, hopelessness, and mood swings. It is important to recognize the signs of depression and seek appropriate support. Engaging in pleasurable activities, maintaining social connections, and practicing self-care can help alleviate depressive symptoms.

Cognitive Changes:

Chemotherapy-induced cognitive changes, commonly referred to as "chemo brain," can affect memory, attention, and concentration. Individuals may experience difficulties with multitasking, organization, and word retrieval. Accepting and adapting to these changes can alleviate frustration. Techniques such as utilizing memory aids, establishing routines, and breaking tasks into smaller, manageable steps can help manage cognitive challenges.

Body Image and Self-esteem:

Chemotherapy treatments can impact body image and self-esteem. Physical changes such as hair loss, weight fluctuations, and skin alterations can affect self-perception and confidence. Seeking support from loved ones, participating in support groups, and engaging in activities that enhance self-expression and self-care can help individuals navigate these challenges. It is important to remember that beauty and self-worth extend beyond physical appearance.

Stress and Coping Mechanisms:

The stress associated with chemotherapy can affect individuals both emotionally and physically. Identifying effective coping mechanisms is essential for managing stress. Techniques such as journaling, engaging in relaxation exercises, practicing mindfulness, and seeking professional counseling can provide outlets for stress reduction. Engaging in activities that bring joy, such as hobbies or creative pursuits, can also serve as healthy coping mechanisms.

Communication and Emotional Support:

Open and honest communication with loved ones and healthcare professionals is crucial. Sharing concerns, fears, and emotions with trusted individuals can provide a sense of relief and support. It is important to express needs and seek emotional support when required. Healthcare professionals can provide information, resources, and referrals to counselors or support groups specializing in emotional support for cancer patients.

Role of Social Support:

Maintaining social connections and seeking support from loved ones play a vital role in emotional well-being. Friends, family, and support groups can offer comfort, understanding, and practical assistance. Engaging in social activities and maintaining regular communication can help individuals feel connected and supported throughout their chemotherapy journey.

Self-care and Wellness:

Prioritizing self-care and wellness is essential for managing the psychological effects of chemotherapy. Engaging in activities that promote relaxation, self-expression, and self-compassion can help foster emotional well-being. These activities may include practicing relaxation techniques, engaging in hobbies, participating in support groups, seeking spiritual guidance, or seeking therapeutic interventions such as massage or acupuncture.

Professional Support:

Seeking professional support from mental health professionals, counselors, or psychologists who specialize in cancer-related issues can be invaluable. These professionals can provide individualized

## Support systems and therapy options

Receiving a diagnosis of cancer and undergoing chemotherapy can be an emotionally challenging journey. Building a strong support system and exploring therapy options can significantly contribute to emotional well-being and help individuals navigate the psychological impact of chemotherapy. This chapter explores the importance of support systems and therapy options and provides insights into the various resources available to individuals undergoing chemotherapy.

Importance of Support Systems:

Having a robust support system is crucial during chemotherapy. Loved ones, friends, and support groups provide emotional comfort, understanding, and encouragement. They can be a source of strength and provide a listening ear during difficult times. Support systems can offer practical assistance with daily tasks, accompany individuals to medical appointments, and provide respite when needed.

Family and Friends:

Family members and close friends often form the primary support network for individuals undergoing chemotherapy. They can provide emotional support, help manage daily responsibilities, and offer a sense of normalcy. Maintaining open lines of communication with loved ones can foster understanding and create an environment where individuals feel safe expressing their emotions and concerns.

Support Groups:

Support groups specifically tailored to cancer patients can offer a unique space for individuals to connect with others who understand their experiences. Sharing stories, insights, and coping strategies with fellow patients can provide a sense of camaraderie and validation. Support groups may be facilitated by healthcare professionals or offered through cancer support organizations.

Online Communities:

In the digital age, online communities have emerged as valuable platforms for individuals undergoing chemotherapy to connect with others facing similar challenges. Online forums and social media groups can provide a space for sharing experiences, seeking advice, and finding emotional support. It is important to engage in reputable and moderated platforms to ensure a safe and supportive environment.

Professional Counseling:

Professional counseling or psychotherapy can be a valuable resource for individuals navigating the emotional impact of chemotherapy. Mental health professionals can provide a safe and confidential space to discuss fears, concerns, and emotional challenges. They offer guidance, coping strategies, and interventions to promote emotional well-being. Counseling sessions can be conducted individually, with family members, or in group settings.

Cognitive-Behavioral Therapy (CBT):

Cognitive-Behavioral Therapy (CBT) is a widely recognized therapeutic approach that focuses on identifying and modifying negative thought patterns and behaviors. CBT can help individuals undergoing chemotherapy develop effective coping mechanisms, challenge negative beliefs, and cultivate resilience. It equips individuals with practical tools to manage anxiety, depression, and stress.

Mindfulness-Based Stress Reduction (MBSR):

Mindfulness-Based Stress Reduction (MBSR) is a therapeutic approach that combines mindfulness meditation, gentle movement, and awareness practices. MBSR teaches individuals to cultivate present-moment awareness, reduce stress, and develop coping skills. It can promote emotional well-being and help individuals manage the challenges of chemotherapy with greater resilience.

Art Therapy:

Art therapy involves engaging in creative processes, such as painting, drawing, or sculpting, to promote self-expression and emotional healing. Art therapy provides a non-verbal outlet for individuals to explore their emotions, reduce anxiety, and process their experiences. It can be a valuable therapeutic tool for individuals who find it difficult to express their feelings verbally.

Music Therapy:

Music therapy uses music-based interventions to address emotional, physical, and psychological needs. Listening to or creating music can evoke positive emotions, reduce anxiety, and promote relaxation. Music therapy can be conducted individually or in group settings, and it offers a unique way for individuals to express themselves, find comfort, and enhance their well-being.

Integrative Therapies:

Integrative therapies, such as massage therapy, acupuncture, and yoga, can complement traditional medical treatments and support emotional well-being during chemotherapy. These therapies promote relaxation

## Stress management techniques

Chemotherapy treatment can bring about various stressors, including physical discomfort, emotional challenges, and uncertainties about the future. Effectively managing stress is crucial for maintaining emotional well-being and overall quality of life during this period. This chapter explores stress management techniques specifically tailored to individuals undergoing chemotherapy, providing insights into practical strategies for nurturing emotional well-being.

Deep Breathing Exercises:

Deep breathing exercises are simple yet effective techniques for reducing stress and promoting relaxation. They can be practiced anywhere, at any time. One popular method is diaphragmatic breathing, where you inhale deeply through your nose, allowing your abdomen to rise, and then exhale slowly through your mouth. Deep breathing helps activate the body's relaxation response and reduces anxiety and tension.

Progressive Muscle Relaxation (PMR):

Progressive muscle relaxation is a technique that involves tensing and relaxing different muscle groups to achieve a state of deep relaxation. Start by tensing a specific muscle group, such as your shoulders, for a few seconds, and then release the tension while focusing on the feeling of relaxation. Move through your body, progressively relaxing each muscle group. PMR helps release muscle tension and promotes overall relaxation and calmness.

Mindfulness Meditation:

Mindfulness meditation involves focusing your attention on the present moment and accepting it without judgment. Find a quiet space, sit comfortably, and bring your awareness to your breath, bodily sensations, or a specific focal point. Whenever your mind wanders, gently bring it back to the present moment. Mindfulness meditation cultivates a sense of calm, reduces anxiety, and enhances overall well-being.

Guided Imagery:

Guided imagery is a technique that uses the power of the imagination to evoke relaxation and positive emotions. Close your eyes, visualize a peaceful or calming scene, and engage your senses to make the visualization vivid. This technique can transport you to a serene mental space, reducing stress and promoting a sense of well-being. Guided imagery recordings or apps are available to assist with the process.

Journaling:

Journaling provides an outlet for expressing emotions, processing experiences, and gaining insights. Set aside time each day to write freely, without judgment or concern for grammar or structure. Write about your thoughts, feelings, challenges, and victories. Journaling allows you to release pent-up emotions, gain clarity, and document your journey, providing a sense of empowerment and self-reflection.

Engaging in Relaxation Activities:

Engaging in activities that promote relaxation can be an effective stress management technique. Listening to soothing music, taking warm baths, practicing yoga or tai chi, engaging in hobbies, or spending time in nature are all valuable ways to relax and reduce stress. Find activities that bring you joy and peace and incorporate them into your routine regularly.

Seeking Emotional Support:

Building a strong support system and seeking emotional support is vital for managing stress during chemotherapy. Reach out to friends, family members, or support groups who can provide a listening ear, understanding, and empathy. Share your feelings, concerns, and challenges openly. Additionally, consider speaking with a therapist or counselor who can offer professional guidance and support.

Time Management:

Managing time effectively can reduce stress and create a sense of control. Prioritize your tasks and break them down into smaller, manageable steps. Delegate responsibilities when possible and learn to say no to non-essential commitments. Creating a schedule and setting realistic expectations can help reduce feelings of overwhelm and promote a sense of achievement.

Physical Activity:

Engaging in regular physical activity has numerous benefits for both physical and emotional well-being. Consult with your healthcare team to determine suitable activities based on your health status. Light exercises such as walking, gentle stretching, or yoga can help reduce stress, increase endorph

Chapter Eight

# Chemotherapy and Hair Loss

One of the most well-known and visible side effects of chemotherapy is hair loss. For many individuals undergoing cancer treatment, the prospect of losing their hair can be emotionally challenging. Understanding the process of chemotherapy-induced hair loss and learning coping strategies can help individuals navigate this aspect of their treatment journey with greater confidence and resilience. This chapter explores the relationship between chemotherapy and hair loss, providing factual information and practical tips for coping with this temporary change.

The Mechanism of Hair Loss:

Chemotherapy drugs target rapidly dividing cells, including cancer cells, but they can also affect healthy cells in the body, including hair follicles. As a result, the hair growth cycle is disrupted, leading to hair loss. The extent and pattern of hair loss vary depending on the type and dosage of chemotherapy drugs, as well as individual factors such as age and overall health.

When Does Hair Loss Occur?

Hair loss usually begins a few weeks after starting chemotherapy treatment. Some individuals experience gradual thinning, while others may lose their hair more rapidly. Hair loss can affect the scalp, eyebrows, eyelashes, and other body hair. It is important to note that not all chemotherapy drugs cause hair loss, and the degree of hair loss can vary.

Preparing for Hair Loss:

Knowing in advance that hair loss is likely to occur can help individuals better prepare for the change. Consider discussing hair loss with your healthcare team before starting treatment. This will allow you to gather information, ask questions, and explore options for managing and coping with hair loss.

Coping with Hair Loss:

Although hair loss can be emotionally challenging, it is essential to remember that it is a temporary side effect of chemotherapy. Here are some coping strategies:

2. a. Consider a New Hairstyle: Before hair loss begins, consider getting a new haircut or hairstyle that can help you transition more comfortably. Opting for shorter hairstyles or gradually reducing the length can make the transition less abrupt.

3. b. Experiment with Head Coverings: Many individuals choose to wear head coverings such as wigs, scarves, hats, or turbans during hair loss. Explore different styles, materials, and colors to find options that feel comfortable and reflect your personal style. Some cancer centers offer resources and assistance in finding suitable head coverings.

4. c. Embrace Your Baldness: Some individuals choose not to cover their heads during hair loss and embrace their baldness. This can be a liberating and empowering choice. If you decide to go bald, consider using sunscreen or wearing a hat to protect your scalp from the sun.

5. d. Care for Your Scalp: Taking care of your scalp is important during hair loss. Keep your scalp clean and moisturized. Use gentle products and avoid harsh chemicals or hot styling tools that may further irritate the scalp.

6. e. Protect Your Hair Follicles: To minimize damage to your hair follicles during chemotherapy, avoid heat styling, hair dyes, and harsh hair products. Be gentle when washing and brushing your hair. Use a wide-toothed comb or a soft brush to prevent unnecessary hair breakage.

7. f. Talk About Your Feelings: Hair loss can evoke a range of emotions. It is important to talk openly about your feelings with supportive family members, friends, or support groups. Sharing your experiences can provide validation, support, and practical tips from others who have gone through similar situations.

Wig Selection and Care:

If you decide to wear a wig during hair loss, take the time to find a wig that suits your preferences and needs. Consider visiting a wig specialist who can help you find the right style, color, and fit. Synthetic wigs are low-maintenance and can be worn immediately, while human hair wigs offer a more natural appearance but

## Why hair loss occurs

Hair loss is a well-known side effect of chemotherapy, causing emotional distress for many individuals undergoing cancer treatment. Understanding the mechanism behind chemotherapy-induced hair loss can help individuals cope with this temporary change more effectively. This chapter explores why hair loss occurs during chemotherapy, shedding light on the physiological process and providing factual information to demystify this aspect of cancer treatment.

Impact on Hair Follicles:

Chemotherapy drugs are designed to target rapidly dividing cells, including cancer cells. Unfortunately, they can also affect other rapidly dividing cells in the body, such as those found in hair follicles. Hair follicles are responsible for producing hair, and they undergo a cycle of growth, rest, and shedding. Chemotherapy disrupts this cycle, leading to hair loss.

Timing of Hair Loss:

Hair loss usually begins a few weeks after starting chemotherapy treatment. The specific timing can vary depending on the type and dosage of chemotherapy drugs used, as well as individual factors such as age, overall health, and the specific cancer being treated. Hair loss may occur gradually or more rapidly, and it can affect the scalp, eyebrows, eyelashes, and body hair.

Different Chemotherapy Drugs:

Not all chemotherapy drugs cause hair loss. Some drugs have a higher likelihood of causing hair loss than others. For example, drugs known as "anthracyclines" (such as doxorubicin) and "taxanes" (such as paclitaxel) commonly result in hair loss. However, the extent and pattern of hair loss can still vary depending on the specific drug regimen and the individual's unique response to treatment.

Impact on Hair Growth Cycle:

2. To understand why hair loss occurs, it's important to recognize the natural hair growth cycle. The hair growth cycle consists of three phases: anagen, catagen, and telogen.

3. Anagen Phase: This is the active growth phase, during which hair follicles produce new hair. The length of the anagen phase determines the length of the hair.

4. Catagen Phase: In this transitional phase, hair follicles shrink and detach from the blood supply, preparing for the next phase.

5. Telogen Phase: Also known as the resting phase, the telogen phase is when the hair follicles are inactive. Eventually, the old hair is shed, making way for new hair growth.

Chemotherapy drugs primarily target cells in the active growth phase (anagen phase), causing the hair follicles to enter the telogen phase prematurely. This disrupts the normal hair growth cycle and leads to hair loss.

Temporary Nature of Hair Loss:

It is important to note that chemotherapy-induced hair loss is usually temporary. Once treatment is completed, the hair follicles gradually recover, and hair regrowth typically begins within a few months. However, the regrowth process may vary among individuals. The texture, color, and thickness of the regrown hair may also differ from the original hair.

Psychological Impact:

Hair loss can have a significant psychological impact on individuals undergoing chemotherapy. It is a visible reminder of their illness and treatment, potentially affecting self-esteem, body image, and overall well-being. Understanding the temporary nature of hair loss and exploring coping strategies can help individuals navigate this aspect of their treatment journey with greater confidence and resilience.

Coping with Hair Loss:

There are various coping strategies individuals can employ to manage hair loss:

6. Wig Selection: Some individuals choose to wear wigs to maintain their appearance and confidence during treatment. Wig specialists can help individuals find wigs that match their natural hair color, style, and comfort level.

7. Head Coverings: Scarves, hats, turbans, and caps are popular alternatives to wigs. They provide practical and fashionable options to cover

## Coping with hair loss

Hair loss is a common side effect of chemotherapy that can significantly impact the emotional well-being of individuals undergoing cancer treatment. Coping with hair loss requires emotional resilience, support, and practical strategies to maintain confidence and embrace change. This chapter explores various ways to cope with hair loss during chemotherapy, providing factual information and practical tips for navigating this aspect of the treatment journey.

Understanding Hair Loss:

Understanding the mechanism and temporary nature of chemotherapy-induced hair loss can help individuals cope with the emotional challenges. It is important to remember that hair loss is a result of the impact of chemotherapy on rapidly dividing cells, including hair follicles. Knowing that hair will eventually regrow after treatment can provide reassurance and alleviate concerns about permanent hair loss.

Self-expression through Head Coverings:

Choosing head coverings is a popular option for individuals experiencing hair loss. Scarves, hats, turbans, and caps can provide comfort, style, and privacy. Experiment with different styles, materials, and colors to find head coverings that suit your personal taste and comfort level. Online tutorials and local cancer support organizations often provide guidance on various wrapping techniques and creative ways to wear head coverings.

Wigs as a Confidence Boost:

Wigs offer an opportunity to maintain a familiar appearance and regain a sense of normalcy. Consult with a wig specialist to find a wig that matches your natural hair color, style, and comfort requirements. Synthetic wigs are often more affordable and low-maintenance, while human hair wigs provide a more natural look and versatility. Proper wig care, including regular cleaning and styling, ensures longevity and a natural appearance.

Embracing Baldness:

Some individuals choose not to wear head coverings or wigs and embrace their baldness confidently. Going bald can be an empowering choice that eliminates the need for additional accessories or maintenance. Emphasize self-acceptance, celebrate the strength of your journey, and remember that bald is beautiful. Protecting the scalp from the sun with sunscreen or hats is important during this time.

Hair and Scalp Care:

Taking care of the scalp and any remaining hair can help maintain comfort and promote a healthy environment for future hair regrowth. Gently cleanse the scalp with mild shampoos or cleansers, avoiding harsh chemicals or excessive rubbing. Moisturize the scalp with gentle lotions or oils to prevent dryness and irritation. Protect the scalp from extreme temperatures, such as cold weather or direct sunlight.

Make-up and Accessories:

Enhancing other aspects of your appearance can help shift the focus away from hair loss. Experiment with make-up techniques to highlight your best features and boost your confidence. Consider using eyebrow pencils or powders to define and shape eyebrows, false eyelashes to add volume, and colorful scarves or statement earrings to draw attention to your face.

These small touches can make a significant difference in how you perceive yourself.

Support from Loved Ones:

Openly communicate with your loved ones about your feelings and concerns regarding hair loss. Share your experience and allow them to offer support and understanding. Engaging in honest conversations helps foster a supportive environment where you can freely express your emotions. Loved ones can provide encouragement, empathy, and reassurance throughout the process.

Support Groups:

Joining support groups or connecting with individuals who have gone through similar experiences can provide a sense of belonging and understanding. Sharing stories, advice, and coping strategies with others facing hair loss can be empowering and comforting. Support groups can be found online or through local cancer support organizations.

Self-care and Self-Expression:

Focus on self-care and activities that bring joy and boost your self-confidence. Engage in hobbies, exercise, meditate, practice mindfulness, or indulge in

## Hair regrowth and care after treatment

After completing chemotherapy treatment, many individuals look forward to the regrowth of their hair. Understanding the process of hair regrowth and adopting proper care practices can help individuals navigate this phase with confidence and support the health of their new hair. This chapter explores the process of hair regrowth after chemotherapy and provides factual information and practical tips for caring for new hair and embracing the changes.

Hair Regrowth Timeline:

Hair regrowth occurs gradually after chemotherapy treatment. It is important to note that the regrowth timeline can vary among individuals. In general, hair starts to regrow within a few weeks to a couple of months after the completion of chemotherapy. Initially, the new hair may be fine, soft, and different in texture and color compared to the original hair. Over time, it will gradually regain its normal characteristics.

Patience and Acceptance:

It is essential to approach hair regrowth with patience and acceptance. The regrowth process takes time, and the appearance of new hair may be different from what you were accustomed to. Embrace the changes and be patient as your hair gradually returns to its pre-treatment state. Remember that regrowth is a positive sign of recovery and a new chapter in your journey.

Gentle Hair Care:

While your new hair is growing, it is important to adopt gentle hair care practices to promote its health and minimize damage. Avoid harsh chemicals, excessive heat styling, and tight hairstyles that can strain the hair follicles. Use mild shampoos and conditioners specifically formulated for sensitive or damaged hair. Pat dry your hair gently with a soft towel rather than rubbing vigorously.

Regular Trims:

Although it may seem counterintuitive, getting regular trims can actually benefit hair regrowth. Trimming the ends of your hair every six to eight weeks helps remove split ends and prevents breakage, allowing your hair to grow longer and stronger. Consult with a professional hairstylist to determine the most appropriate trimming schedule for your hair type and growth rate.

Balanced Diet and Nutritional Support:

A balanced diet plays a vital role in supporting hair health and growth. Ensure you are getting an adequate intake of essential nutrients, including protein, vitamins (particularly vitamin D, E, and B vitamins), minerals (such as iron and zinc), and omega-3 fatty acids. Consult with a healthcare professional or registered dietitian to address any specific nutritional concerns or deficiencies.

Scalp Massage:

Massaging the scalp can help stimulate blood circulation to the hair follicles, promoting hair growth. Gently massage your scalp using your fingertips in a circular motion for a few minutes each day. This technique not only supports hair regrowth but also provides a relaxing experience and relieves tension.

Avoid Overwashing:

While maintaining cleanliness is important, overwashing your hair can strip away its natural oils, leading to dryness and potential damage. Aim to wash your hair every two to three days or as recommended by your hairstylist or healthcare professional. Use lukewarm water and gentle shampoo, and consider incorporating a moisturizing conditioner to keep your hair hydrated.

Protecting Your Hair:

Protecting your hair from environmental stressors and damage is crucial for its health and regrowth. Avoid excessive exposure to the sun's harmful UV rays by wearing hats or using sunscreen on your scalp. Minimize the use of heated styling tools, such as straighteners and curling irons, as they can cause damage to the hair shaft. If you do use heat styling tools, apply a heat protectant product beforehand.

Embrace Styling Options:

During the regrowth phase, experiment with different hairstyles and styling options to embrace the changes and boost your confidence. Try out new hair accessories, experiment

Chapter Nine

# Chemotherapy and Fertility

Chemotherapy, a vital treatment for cancer, can have significant implications for fertility. Understanding the impact of chemotherapy on reproductive health and exploring available options is crucial for individuals who wish to preserve their fertility or plan for future family-building. This chapter explores the relationship between chemotherapy and fertility, providing factual information and insights into the options and considerations for individuals undergoing cancer treatment.

Impact on Fertility:

Chemotherapy drugs are designed to target rapidly dividing cells, including cancer cells. Unfortunately, they can also affect healthy cells, including those involved in reproductive function. The impact of chemotherapy on fertility depends on various factors, such as the type, dosage, and duration of treatment, as well as the individual's age, overall health, and reproductive health prior to treatment.

Temporary or Permanent Infertility:

Chemotherapy can cause temporary or permanent infertility. Temporary infertility occurs when the menstrual cycle is disrupted during treatment, but fertility is restored once the treatment is completed. Permanent infertility may occur when chemotherapy damages the ovaries or testes, affecting the production of eggs or sperm.

Factors Influencing Fertility Impact:

Several factors contribute to the impact of chemotherapy on fertility:

2. Age: Fertility decreases with age, and older individuals may have a higher risk of permanent infertility due to chemotherapy.

3. Drug Type and Dosage: Different chemotherapy drugs have varying effects on fertility. Some drugs have a higher likelihood of causing infertility than others. The dosage and duration of treatment also play a role.

4. Reproductive Health Prior to Treatment: The individual's fertility status before treatment, including factors such as ovarian reserve, semen quality, and overall reproductive health, can influence the impact of chemotherapy on fertility.

Fertility Preservation Options for Women:

For women, several fertility preservation options may be available before starting chemotherapy:

5. Egg Freezing: Mature eggs are harvested, frozen, and stored for future use. This process typically involves hormone stimulation and egg retrieval.

6. Embryo Freezing: Eggs are fertilized with sperm to create embryos, which are then frozen and stored for future use. This option requires a partner or the use of donor sperm.

7. Ovarian Tissue Freezing: A surgical procedure is performed to remove a portion of the ovary, which contains immature eggs. The tissue is frozen and can be re-implanted or used for egg retrieval in the future.

Fertility Preservation Options for Men:

For men, fertility preservation options include:

8. Sperm Banking: Semen samples are collected and frozen for future use. This option is relatively straightforward and non-invasive.

Timing of Fertility Preservation:

Timing is critical when considering fertility preservation options. It is recommended to discuss fertility preservation with a reproductive specialist before starting chemotherapy. Some fertility preservation procedures may need to be completed before treatment begins, while others can be performed during treatment. The individual's overall health and treatment timeline should be considered when determining the most suitable approach.

Oncofertility Specialists:

Oncofertility specialists are healthcare professionals who specialize in fertility preservation for individuals undergoing cancer treatment. They can provide personalized guidance, discuss available options, and address any concerns related to fertility preservation.

Future Fertility Considerations:

Even if fertility preservation is not pursued, it is important to discuss future fertility considerations with a healthcare provider. Depending on the treatment and its impact on fertility, alternative family-building options such as adoption, surrogacy, or using donor gametes may be explored. Open communication with a healthcare team and counseling support can help individuals make informed decisions about their reproductive options.

Emotional Support and Counseling:

The emotional impact of infertility and the prospect of losing fertility can be significant. It is crucial to seek emotional support and counseling to navigate the complex emotions that may arise

## Chemotherapy's impact on fertility

Chemotherapy, a vital treatment for cancer, can have a significant impact on fertility. Understanding how chemotherapy affects fertility and exploring available options is crucial for individuals who wish to preserve their fertility or plan for future family-building. This chapter explores the relationship between chemotherapy and fertility, providing factual information and insights into the impact of chemotherapy on reproductive health.

Mechanism of Impact:

Chemotherapy drugs are designed to target and destroy rapidly dividing cells, including cancer cells. Unfortunately, they can also affect healthy cells in the body, including those involved in reproductive function. The impact of chemotherapy on fertility depends on various factors, such as the specific drugs used, the dosage and duration of treatment, the individual's age, and their reproductive health prior to treatment.

Impact on Women's Fertility:

Chemotherapy can affect women's fertility in different ways:

2. Ovarian Function: Chemotherapy drugs can damage the ovaries, leading to a decrease in the number of eggs and a decline in ovarian function. This can result in menstrual irregularities, premature menopause, or infertility.

3. Ovarian Reserve: Chemotherapy can deplete the ovarian reserve, which refers to the number and quality of eggs a woman has in her ovaries. A decrease in ovarian reserve can affect fertility and the chances of successful conception in the future.

4. Menstrual Irregularities: Chemotherapy can cause temporary or permanent disruptions in the menstrual cycle, including irregular periods, absence of periods, or early menopause.

Impact on Men's Fertility:

Chemotherapy can also impact men's fertility in various ways:

5. Sperm Production: Chemotherapy drugs can impair sperm production and quality, leading to a decrease in sperm count, motility, and morphology.

6. Hormonal Imbalance: Chemotherapy can disrupt hormone levels, affecting the normal functioning of the testes and sperm production.

Fertility Preservation Options for Women:

For women, several fertility preservation options may be available before starting chemotherapy:

7. Egg Freezing: Mature eggs are harvested, frozen, and stored for future use. This process typically involves hormone stimulation and egg retrieval.

8. Embryo Freezing: Eggs are fertilized with sperm to create embryos, which are then frozen and stored for future use. This option requires a partner or the use of donor sperm.

9. Ovarian Tissue Freezing: A surgical procedure is performed to remove a portion of the ovary, which contains immature eggs. The tissue is frozen and can be re-implanted or used for egg retrieval in the future.

Fertility Preservation Options for Men:

For men, fertility preservation options include:

10. Sperm Banking: Semen samples are collected and frozen for future use. This option is relatively straightforward and non-invasive.

Timing of Fertility Preservation:

Timing is crucial when considering fertility preservation options. It is recommended to discuss fertility preservation with a reproductive specialist before starting chemotherapy. Some fertility preservation procedures may need to be completed before treatment begins, while others can be performed during treatment. The individual's overall health and treatment timeline should be considered when determining the most suitable approach.

Oncofertility Specialists:

Oncofertility specialists are healthcare professionals who specialize in fertility preservation for individuals undergoing cancer treatment. They can provide personalized guidance, discuss available options, and address any concerns related to fertility preservation.

Fertility after Chemotherapy:

The impact of chemotherapy on fertility varies among individuals. While some individuals may experience temporary fertility issues that resolve after treatment, others may face permanent infertility. It is important to discuss fertility concerns with a healthcare provider to understand the potential impact of chemotherapy on future fertility.

Alternatives for Family-Building:

For individuals who experience permanent infertility or choose not to pursue fertility

## Fertility preservation options

For individuals undergoing chemotherapy, fertility preservation options offer hope for future family-building. The impact of chemotherapy on reproductive health can be significant, making it essential to explore available options before starting treatment. This chapter explores various fertility preservation options, providing factual information and insights into empowering individuals during chemotherapy.

Egg Freezing:

Egg freezing, also known as oocyte cryopreservation, is a popular option for women seeking fertility preservation. It involves the extraction and freezing of mature eggs for future use. Before starting chemotherapy, women undergo ovarian stimulation through hormone injections to encourage multiple eggs to develop. Once the eggs reach maturity, they are retrieved and cryopreserved. In the future, when ready to conceive, the eggs can be thawed, fertilized with sperm through in vitro fertilization (IVF), and transferred to the uterus.

Embryo Freezing:

Embryo freezing is an option for women in a committed relationship or using donor sperm. In this process, eggs are retrieved through ovarian stimulation, and sperm is collected from the partner or a sperm donor. The eggs are fertilized with the sperm, and resulting embryos are cryopreserved for future use. When ready to conceive, the embryos are thawed and transferred to the uterus.

Ovarian Tissue Freezing:

Ovarian tissue freezing is an innovative technique for women who cannot undergo ovarian stimulation or have limited time before starting chemotherapy. It involves the surgical removal of a portion of the ovary containing immature eggs. The tissue is then cryopreserved for future use. In the future, the ovarian tissue can be re-implanted, or the eggs can be retrieved from the tissue and used for IVF.

Sperm Banking:

Sperm banking is a straightforward option for men seeking fertility preservation. Semen samples are collected and frozen for future use. The samples can be stored for an extended period without significant loss in quality. When ready to conceive, the samples can be thawed and used for insemination or IVF.

Preimplantation Genetic Testing (PGT):

Preimplantation genetic testing is a technique that can be used in conjunction with embryo freezing. PGT allows for the screening of embryos for genetic abnormalities before transfer to the uterus. This testing can provide individuals with additional information about the embryos' genetic health, increasing the chances of a successful pregnancy.

GnRH Agonist:

Gonadotropin-releasing hormone (GnRH) agonists, such as leuprolide, can be used as an adjunct therapy to protect the ovaries during chemotherapy. These medications work by temporarily suppressing ovarian function, reducing the potential damage caused by chemotherapy drugs. GnRH agonists can help preserve fertility, particularly in women who are unable to undergo egg or embryo freezing.

Consultation with Fertility Specialists:

When considering fertility preservation options, it is crucial to consult with fertility specialists or reproductive endocrinologists who have experience in oncofertility. These specialists can assess individual circumstances, discuss available options, and tailor a preservation plan that aligns with personal goals and medical considerations.

Timing of Fertility Preservation:

The timing of fertility preservation is critical. Ideally, discussions about fertility preservation should occur before starting chemotherapy to maximize the available options. However, fertility preservation may still be possible during chemotherapy in some cases. It is important to remember that fertility preservation decisions are individualized, and a multidisciplinary approach involving oncologists, fertility specialists, and support from counseling professionals is beneficial.

Emotional Support and Counseling:

Decisions regarding fertility preservation can evoke a range of emotions, including anxiety, grief, and uncertainty. Seeking emotional support and counseling throughout the process is essential. Counselors, therapists, or support groups can provide guidance,

## Family planning and support

For individuals undergoing chemotherapy, family planning and support are vital considerations that go beyond medical treatment. The impact of chemotherapy on fertility and the emotional journey that accompanies it can significantly influence decisions about building a family. This chapter explores family planning options and the importance of support during chemotherapy, providing factual information and insights into empowering individuals on their journey.

Pre-treatment Discussions:

Early discussions with healthcare providers regarding family planning can provide individuals with a clear understanding of the potential impact of chemotherapy on fertility. It is essential to communicate personal goals and desires regarding family-building to ensure that appropriate fertility preservation options are explored before treatment begins.

Fertility Preservation:

Fertility preservation options, such as egg freezing, embryo freezing, sperm banking, or ovarian tissue freezing, can provide hope for future family-building. These techniques allow individuals to preserve their reproductive cells or tissue for use after completing chemotherapy. Exploring these options with the guidance of fertility specialists can provide a sense of control and peace of mind during the treatment process.

Alternatives to Biological Parenthood:

For individuals unable to pursue fertility preservation or experiencing permanent infertility due to chemotherapy, exploring alternative paths to parenthood can be empowering. Adoption, surrogacy, or using donor gametes (eggs or sperm) are options that offer the opportunity to build a family and experience the joys of parenthood. Seeking information and support from adoption agencies, surrogacy organizations, or reproductive counseling services can help individuals navigate these alternatives.

Emotional Support:

The emotional journey of undergoing chemotherapy and facing potential fertility challenges requires a strong support system. Engaging with family, friends, support groups, or professional counselors can provide a safe space to express emotions, seek guidance, and share experiences. These avenues for support can help individuals process their feelings, alleviate anxiety, and develop coping mechanisms during this challenging time.

Partner and Family Involvement:

Including partners and family members in discussions about family planning and support can foster a sense of unity and shared decision-making. Open and honest communication with loved ones allows for mutual understanding, emotional support, and collective problem-solving. It is important to ensure that everyone involved feels heard, respected, and included in the decision-making process.

Oncofertility Programs:

Oncofertility programs specialize in providing comprehensive support for individuals facing fertility challenges due to cancer treatment. These programs offer a multidisciplinary approach, combining the expertise of oncologists, fertility specialists, and mental health professionals. Oncofertility programs can provide guidance on fertility preservation options, emotional support, and resources for family planning during and after chemotherapy.

Financial Considerations:

Family planning options and fertility preservation can involve financial implications. It is essential to consider the costs associated with fertility preservation procedures, such as consultations, medications, and storage fees. Exploring available financial resources, insurance coverage, and potential grants or assistance programs can help individuals make informed decisions and alleviate financial stress.

Future Family-Building Timeline:

Timing is a crucial factor in family planning. The impact of chemotherapy on fertility, the recovery process, and individual circumstances should be taken into account when determining the appropriate time to pursue family-building options. Discussing the timeline with healthcare providers, fertility specialists, and support professionals can help create a realistic plan that aligns with personal goals and medical considerations.

Counseling and Decision-Making:

Navigating family planning decisions during chemotherapy can be overwhelming. Seeking counseling support can assist individuals in exploring their values, clarifying priorities, and making informed decisions about family-building options. Counseling professionals can provide guidance, help weigh the pros and cons of different paths, and facilitate the decision-making process in a supportive and non-judgmental environment.

Resilience and Self-Care:

Maintaining resilience and prioritizing

Chapter Ten

# Financial Considerations and Resources

The financial impact of chemotherapy extends beyond medical expenses, often encompassing costs associated with medications, supportive care, and lifestyle adjustments. Understanding the financial considerations and available resources can help individuals navigate the financial challenges associated with chemotherapy. This chapter explores the financial aspects of chemotherapy, providing factual information and insights into accessing resources and managing costs effectively.

Medical Expenses:

Chemotherapy treatments involve various medical expenses, including consultations, diagnostic tests, chemotherapy drugs, and hospital stays. These costs can vary depending on the specific treatment regimen, healthcare provider, and insurance coverage. It is essential to consult with healthcare providers and insurance representatives to understand the expected costs and coverage associated with chemotherapy.

Insurance Coverage:

Reviewing health insurance policies is crucial to understand coverage details for chemotherapy. Different insurance plans may have varying levels of coverage for chemotherapy drugs, hospital stays, and supportive care. Familiarize yourself with the terms and limitations of your insurance policy, such as deductibles, copayments, and maximum coverage limits.

Contacting the insurance provider or utilizing the services of a patient advocate can help clarify coverage and address any concerns.

Out-of-Pocket Expenses:

Even with insurance coverage, individuals may still encounter out-of-pocket expenses. These can include copayments, deductibles, and costs for non-covered services or medications. Budgeting for these expenses and planning ahead can help manage the financial burden associated with chemotherapy. Exploring available financial assistance programs, grants, and discounts from pharmaceutical companies or charitable organizations can alleviate some of the out-of-pocket costs.

Prescription Medication Costs:

Chemotherapy drugs can be expensive, and copayments or coinsurance for these medications can add up quickly. It is essential to communicate with healthcare providers about cost concerns and explore options for accessing affordable medications. Some pharmaceutical companies offer patient assistance programs or copay assistance cards that can reduce the financial burden of chemotherapy drugs.

Supportive Care Expenses:

Supportive care, such as medications for managing side effects, nutritional supplements, or complementary therapies, may also contribute to the overall cost of chemotherapy. These expenses can vary depending on individual needs and preferences. Discussing supportive care options with healthcare providers and exploring generic alternatives or cost-saving measures can help minimize these expenses.

Lifestyle Adjustments:

Chemotherapy treatment may necessitate lifestyle adjustments, such as transportation to and from medical appointments, dietary changes, or modifications to work schedules. These adjustments can have financial implications, such as transportation costs or the need for meal deliveries. Planning for these changes, exploring available resources within the community, and discussing potential workplace accommodations with employers can help manage associated costs.

Financial Assistance Programs:

Various financial assistance programs are available to support individuals undergoing chemotherapy. These programs can help cover medical expenses, prescription costs, and other related costs. Non-profit organizations, government agencies, and cancer-specific foundations often offer financial assistance or grants. Seeking information from healthcare providers, social workers, or patient advocacy groups can help identify relevant programs and resources.

Patient Assistance Programs:

Pharmaceutical companies may provide patient assistance programs that offer reduced-cost or free medications to individuals who meet specific eligibility criteria. These programs can significantly alleviate the financial burden of chemotherapy drugs. Researching and contacting pharmaceutical companies or utilizing online resources that aggregate information about patient assistance programs can provide access to these resources.

Social Work and Financial Counseling:

Hospitals and cancer centers often have social workers or financial counselors who can provide guidance on financial matters. These professionals can help individuals understand the available resources, navigate insurance-related issues, and explore financial assistance programs. They can also assist in applying for grants, accessing charitable organizations, or exploring options for financial support.

Budgeting and Financial Planning:

Creating a budget and financial plan is essential when undergoing chemotherapy.

## The cost of chemotherapy

Chemotherapy is a critical component of cancer treatment, but its cost extends beyond medical expenses, often posing financial challenges for individuals and their families. Understanding the cost of chemotherapy and exploring available resources can help individuals navigate the financial burden associated with this essential therapy. This chapter explores the various factors that contribute to the cost of chemotherapy, providing factual information and insights into managing expenses effectively.

Medication Costs:

Chemotherapy drugs play a significant role in the cost of treatment. These drugs can be expensive due to the research, development, and production involved. The cost of chemotherapy drugs varies depending on the specific drugs used, dosage requirements, treatment duration, and whether the drugs are administered orally or intravenously. It is important to consult with healthcare providers and insurance representatives to understand the costs associated with specific chemotherapy drugs.

Treatment Setting:

The location and setting of chemotherapy treatment can impact its cost. Chemotherapy can be administered in various settings, including hospitals, outpatient clinics, and specialized cancer centers. The cost of treatment may vary depending on the facility and associated services. Outpatient clinics or infusion centers generally have lower costs compared to hospital-based treatments. Understanding the different options available and their associated costs can help individuals make informed decisions.

Frequency and Duration of Treatment:

The frequency and duration of chemotherapy treatment contribute to its cost. Treatment plans vary depending on the type and stage of cancer, as well as individual factors. Some individuals may require several rounds of chemotherapy administered over a few months, while others may undergo treatment for an extended period. Longer treatment durations and frequent administration can increase the overall cost of chemotherapy.

Supportive Care and Medications:

Supportive care during chemotherapy includes medications, laboratory tests, and other interventions to manage side effects and ensure the best possible outcomes. These additional expenses, such as anti-nausea medications, pain management drugs, and blood tests, contribute to the overall cost of treatment. It is important to discuss supportive care options with healthcare providers to understand the associated costs and explore ways to manage expenses effectively.

Diagnostic Tests and Imaging:

Diagnostic tests and imaging play a crucial role in cancer diagnosis, staging, and monitoring during chemotherapy. These tests, including blood work, biopsies, scans, and imaging studies, contribute to the overall cost of treatment. The frequency and type of tests required vary depending on the individual's condition and treatment plan. It is important to work closely with healthcare providers to understand the necessity of these tests and their associated costs.

Health Insurance Coverage:

Health insurance coverage plays a significant role in managing the cost of chemotherapy. The extent of coverage depends on the specific insurance policy, including factors such as deductibles, copayments, and maximum coverage limits. It is important to review insurance policies carefully, understand the terms and limitations, and communicate with insurance representatives to clarify coverage details related to chemotherapy.

Out-of-Pocket Expenses:

Despite insurance coverage, individuals undergoing chemotherapy may encounter out-of-pocket expenses. These expenses can include deductibles, copayments, and costs associated with non-covered services or medications. It is important to budget for these expenses and plan accordingly. Exploring available financial assistance programs, grants, and discounts from pharmaceutical companies or charitable organizations can help manage the financial burden of out-of-pocket costs.

Financial Assistance Programs:

Various financial assistance programs are available to support individuals undergoing chemotherapy. Non-profit organizations, government agencies, and cancer-specific foundations offer financial assistance or grants to help cover medical expenses, medication costs, transportation expenses, and other related costs. Researching and reaching out to these organizations can provide access to valuable resources and support.

Patient Assistance Programs:

Pharmaceutical companies may provide patient assistance programs that offer reduced-cost or free medications to individuals who meet specific eligibility criteria

## Insurance coverage and assistance

When undergoing chemotherapy, understanding insurance coverage and available assistance programs is crucial for managing the financial burden associated with cancer treatment. Insurance coverage plays a significant role in determining the out-of-pocket costs of chemotherapy, while assistance programs provide valuable resources and support. This chapter explores the importance of insurance coverage and the availability of assistance programs, providing factual information and insights into navigating financial support during chemotherapy.

Understanding Insurance Coverage:

Understanding the details of insurance coverage is essential when it comes to managing the cost of chemotherapy. Here are key aspects to consider:

2. Insurance Policy: Review your health insurance policy to understand the specific terms, coverage limits, and benefits related to chemotherapy treatment. Pay attention to deductible amounts, copayments, coinsurance, and maximum coverage limits.

3. Provider Network: Determine if your healthcare providers, including oncologists and chemotherapy infusion centers, are in-network or out-of-network. In-network providers typically have negotiated rates with the insurance company, resulting in lower out-of-pocket costs.

4. Prior Authorization: Confirm whether prior authorization is required for chemotherapy treatment. This step involves obtaining approval from the insurance company before receiving certain treatments or medications. Failure to obtain prior authorization can result in denial of coverage or higher costs.

5. Formulary and Tiered Medications: Understand the formulary of your insurance plan, which is the list of medications covered by the plan. Chemotherapy drugs may be classified into different tiers, with different levels of coverage and associated costs. Ensure that the prescribed medications are covered and determine if there are any lower-cost alternatives.

6. Appeals Process: Familiarize yourself with the appeals process provided by your insurance company. If a claim is denied or coverage is limited, you have the right to appeal the decision. Understanding this process can help you navigate potential coverage issues.

Financial Assistance Programs:

Financial assistance programs can provide valuable support to individuals undergoing chemotherapy. Here are some resources to explore:

7. Pharmaceutical Patient Assistance Programs: Many pharmaceutical companies offer patient assistance programs that provide free or reduced-cost medications to eligible individuals. These programs are typically based on income and provide access to chemotherapy drugs at a lower cost or no cost.

8. Non-Profit Organizations: Numerous non-profit organizations focus on assisting individuals with cancer-related expenses. These organizations offer financial assistance for medical bills, transportation costs, housing, and other related expenses. Researching and reaching out to cancer-specific organizations or local support groups can help identify available resources.

9. Government Assistance Programs: Government programs such as Medicaid, Medicare, or state-funded assistance programs can provide financial support for healthcare expenses. These programs have eligibility criteria based on income and other factors. Exploring these options and

understanding the requirements can help individuals access financial assistance during chemotherapy.

10. Charitable Foundations and Grants: Charitable foundations and grants offer financial support to individuals undergoing chemotherapy. These organizations may provide grants for medical expenses, transportation, and supportive care services. Researching cancer-specific foundations and grant opportunities can uncover additional financial support options.

Insurance Navigation Services:

Insurance navigation services or patient advocates can provide guidance and support in navigating insurance-related challenges. These professionals are well-versed in insurance terminology, coverage options, and can assist with understanding insurance policies, filing claims, and resolving coverage issues. Utilizing the services of an insurance navigator or patient advocate can help individuals maximize their insurance benefits and reduce financial stress.

Hospital Financial Counselors:

Many hospitals and cancer centers have financial counselors who specialize in helping patients understand their insurance coverage and navigate the financial aspects of treatment. These counselors can assist in exploring available assistance programs, reviewing insurance claims, and addressing billing concerns. Contacting the financial counselor at the healthcare facility can provide valuable information and guidance regarding financial support options.

Workplace Benefits and Assistance:

Employees undergoing chemotherapy should review their workplace benefits to determine the available support.

## Financial support resources

Chemotherapy treatment can bring about significant financial burdens for individuals and their families. From medical expenses to supportive care costs, managing the financial aspects of chemotherapy can be overwhelming. Fortunately, there are various financial support resources available to help individuals navigate these challenges. This chapter explores the importance of financial support resources and provides factual information and insights into accessing assistance during chemotherapy.

Health Insurance:

Health insurance plays a vital role in managing the cost of chemotherapy. Understanding the coverage provided by your insurance policy is essential. Consider the following:

2. Policy Details: Review your insurance policy to understand the terms, limitations, and benefits related to chemotherapy treatment. Pay attention to copayments, deductibles, coinsurance, and maximum coverage limits.

3. Provider Network: Determine if your healthcare providers, including oncologists and chemotherapy infusion centers, are in-network or out-of-network. In-network providers generally have negotiated rates with the insurance company, resulting in lower out-of-pocket costs.

4. Prior Authorization: Find out if prior authorization is required for chemotherapy treatment. This step involves obtaining approval from the insurance company before receiving certain treatments or medications. Failure to obtain prior authorization can result in denial of coverage or higher costs.

Financial Assistance Programs:

Various financial assistance programs can provide valuable support to individuals undergoing chemotherapy. Explore the following resources:

5. Pharmaceutical Patient Assistance Programs: Many pharmaceutical companies offer patient assistance programs that provide free or reduced-cost medications to eligible individuals. These programs are typically based on income and can help individuals access chemotherapy drugs at a lower cost or no cost.

6. Non-Profit Organizations: Numerous non-profit organizations focus on assisting individuals with cancer-related expenses. These organizations offer financial assistance for medical bills, transportation costs, housing, and other related expenses. Researching and reaching out to cancer-specific organizations or local support groups can help identify available resources.

7. Government Assistance Programs: Government programs such as Medicaid, Medicare, or state-funded assistance programs can provide financial support for healthcare expenses. These programs have eligibility criteria based on income and other factors. Exploring these options and understanding the requirements can help individuals access financial assistance during chemotherapy.

8. Charitable Foundations and Grants: Charitable foundations and grants offer financial support to individuals undergoing chemotherapy. These organizations may provide grants for medical expenses, transportation, and supportive care services. Researching cancer-specific foundations and grant opportunities can uncover additional financial support options.

Hospital Financial Counseling:

Many hospitals and cancer centers have financial counselors who specialize in helping patients understand their insurance coverage and navigate the financial aspects of treatment. These counselors can assist in exploring available assistance programs, reviewing insurance claims, and addressing billing concerns. Contacting the financial counselor at the healthcare facility can provide valuable information and guidance regarding financial support options.

Co-Pay Assistance Programs:

Co-pay assistance programs can help individuals manage the out-of-pocket costs associated with chemotherapy. These programs, often provided by pharmaceutical companies, offer financial assistance to individuals who cannot afford their medication co-payments. Researching co-pay assistance programs related to specific chemotherapy drugs can help reduce the financial burden of treatment.

Cancer-Specific Financial Resources:

Numerous cancer-specific organizations and resources provide financial assistance and support services. These organizations aim to alleviate the financial stress faced by individuals undergoing chemotherapy. They may offer grants, scholarships, transportation assistance, and co-pay assistance for medications. Researching cancer-specific financial resources can uncover valuable options for financial support.

Local Community Support:

Local communities often have resources and support services available to help individuals undergoing chemotherapy. These resources may include local charities, religious organizations, or community-based initiatives that provide financial assistance or supportive services. Reaching out to local community centers, social workers, or patient advocacy groups can provide information on available resources.

Patient Assistance Foundations:

Patient assistance foundations are non-profit organizations that offer financial assistance to

Chapter Eleven

# Chemotherapy and Work or School

Chemotherapy is a crucial component of cancer treatment, but it can pose significant challenges when it comes to managing work or school commitments. The side effects of chemotherapy can impact daily functioning and may require individuals to make adjustments to their work or school schedules. This chapter explores the impact of chemotherapy on work or school, providing factual information and insights into effectively managing treatment and responsibilities.

Communicating with Employers or Educators:

Open and honest communication is key when facing chemotherapy treatment while employed or attending school. It is important to inform employers or educators about the diagnosis and treatment plan as soon as possible. Discussing the anticipated schedule, potential side effects, and necessary accommodations can help create a supportive environment and facilitate planning for treatment and work or school responsibilities.

Flexible Work or School Arrangements:

Flexible work or school arrangements can provide individuals undergoing chemotherapy with the necessary flexibility to manage treatment and responsibilities. Some options to consider include:

2. Remote Work or Online Classes: Depending on the nature of the job or educational institution, working remotely or participating in online classes

can provide flexibility in scheduling and reduce the need for travel and physical presence.

3. Adjusted Hours: Modifying work hours or school schedules to accommodate treatment appointments or periods of fatigue can help individuals maintain their work or school commitments while allowing time for rest and recovery.

4. Reduced Workload: In some cases, reducing the workload or adjusting the academic curriculum can alleviate stress and allow individuals to focus on treatment while still progressing in their professional or educational endeavors.

Legal Protections:

Laws and regulations exist to protect individuals facing medical treatments, including chemotherapy, in the workplace or educational setting. Familiarizing oneself with these legal protections can help ensure that individuals receive appropriate accommodations and support. Examples include the Americans with Disabilities Act (ADA) in the United States and similar legislation in other countries.

Taking Time Off:

Depending on the treatment schedule and individual needs, taking time off work or school may be necessary. Medical leave or disability benefits may be available through employer-provided programs, government assistance, or insurance policies. Discussing these options with employers or educational institutions and seeking guidance from human resources or disability services can help navigate the process.

Managing Side Effects:

Chemotherapy can cause various side effects that may impact work or school performance. Some common side effects include fatigue, nausea, cognitive changes, and immune system suppression. Taking steps to manage these side effects can help individuals maintain productivity and well-being:

5. Fatigue Management: Planning for regular rest periods, adjusting work or school schedules to accommodate rest, and prioritizing self-care activities can help manage chemotherapy-related fatigue.

6. Nausea Control: Working with healthcare providers to develop strategies for managing nausea, such as taking anti-nausea medications as prescribed and adjusting eating habits, can help individuals feel more comfortable and maintain productivity.

7. Cognitive Function: Chemotherapy-related cognitive changes, often referred to as "chemo brain," can affect memory, concentration, and multitasking abilities. Employing strategies such as using organizational tools, breaking tasks into manageable segments, and seeking support from colleagues or teachers can help mitigate these challenges.

Workplace or School Support:

Seeking support from colleagues, supervisors, or teachers can be invaluable when balancing chemotherapy treatment and work or school responsibilities:

8. Colleague and Supervisor Understanding: Educating colleagues and supervisors about chemotherapy treatment and its potential impact on work can foster empathy and understanding. Sharing information about treatment schedules, side effects, and necessary accommodations can help create a supportive work environment.

9. Disability or Support Services: Utilizing workplace or educational institution disability services, if available, can provide access to resources and accommodations tailored to individual needs. These services can include flexibility in deadlines, modified workstations, or additional support during challenging periods.

Support from Pe

## Balancing treatment and responsibilities

Chemotherapy treatment is a challenging journey that often requires individuals to navigate the delicate balance between their health needs and various responsibilities. Whether it's managing work, family, or personal commitments, finding harmony amidst chemotherapy treatment can be overwhelming. This chapter explores strategies and insights for effectively balancing treatment and responsibilities, providing factual information and practical tips to empower individuals on their journey.

Prioritize Self-Care:

Self-care is essential when facing the demands of chemotherapy treatment and daily responsibilities. Prioritizing physical and emotional well-being can help individuals maintain their energy, resilience, and overall health. Here are some self-care strategies to consider:

2. Rest and Sleep: Getting enough restorative sleep and allowing time for relaxation and rejuvenation are crucial during chemotherapy. Establishing a regular sleep routine, creating a calming bedtime ritual, and incorporating relaxation techniques, such as meditation or deep breathing exercises, can promote better sleep quality.

3. Nutrition: Eating a balanced diet that includes nutrient-rich foods can support overall health and aid in managing chemotherapy side effects.

Working with a registered dietitian or nutritionist can help individuals identify dietary adjustments to support their specific needs during treatment.

4. Physical Activity: Engaging in gentle exercise or physical activities, as advised by healthcare professionals, can promote overall well-being and help manage fatigue. Incorporating activities like walking, yoga, or tai chi into daily routines can provide physical and mental benefits.

5. Emotional Support: Seeking emotional support through counseling, support groups, or talking with loved ones can provide an outlet for expressing feelings and receiving guidance. Emotional well-being is an integral part of the journey, and acknowledging and addressing emotions is vital.

Communicate and Set Boundaries:

Open and honest communication is key when balancing treatment and responsibilities. Effectively communicating with employers, family members, and friends can help establish boundaries and garner the support needed during this challenging time. Consider the following strategies:

6. Work: Communicate with supervisors and colleagues about treatment schedules, potential side effects, and necessary accommodations. Discuss the possibility of flexible work arrangements, adjusted hours, or workload modifications that can help manage both treatment and work responsibilities effectively.

7. Family and Friends: Share your chemotherapy treatment plan and its potential impact on your daily life with loved ones. Communicate your needs and limitations, and discuss ways they can provide support. Setting boundaries and expressing expectations can help create a supportive network around you.

8. Personal Commitments: Prioritize and evaluate personal commitments, such as social engagements or extracurricular activities, during chemotherapy treatment. Be selective about the activities you choose to participate in and consider rescheduling or delegating tasks when necessary. Remember that it's okay to say "no" and prioritize your well-being.

Time Management and Planning:

Effective time management is crucial for balancing treatment and responsibilities. Planning ahead and organizing tasks can help alleviate stress and create a sense of control. Consider the following strategies:

9. Treatment Schedule: Maintain a calendar or planner to track chemotherapy appointments, follow-up visits, and other medical commitments. Be aware of potential side effects and schedule important activities accordingly, allowing time for rest and recovery.

10. Task Prioritization: Prioritize tasks based on importance and urgency. Focus on essential responsibilities and delegate or postpone non-essential tasks when possible. Break larger tasks into smaller, manageable steps to avoid feeling overwhelmed.

11. Daily Planning: Start each day by reviewing and prioritizing tasks. Create a to-do list and establish a realistic timeline for accomplishing them. Include breaks and self-care activities in your daily schedule to maintain balance and prevent burnout.

12. Support Systems: Lean on the support of family members, friends, or colleagues to help with tasks when needed. Delegate responsibilities, ask for assistance, or consider hiring external help to share the load.

Flexibility and Adapt

## Legal rights and accommodations

When undergoing chemotherapy, individuals have legal rights and protections to ensure they are treated fairly and provided with necessary accommodations in various settings, including the workplace and educational institutions. Understanding these rights and knowing how to navigate legal frameworks can help individuals facing chemotherapy treatment advocate for themselves and receive the support they need. This chapter explores legal rights and accommodations in relation to chemotherapy, providing factual information and insights to empower individuals during their treatment journey.

Americans with Disabilities Act (ADA):

The Americans with Disabilities Act (ADA) is a federal law in the United States that prohibits discrimination against individuals with disabilities, including those facing cancer-related conditions. Key aspects of the ADA include:

2. Definition of Disability: The ADA defines disability as a physical or mental impairment that substantially limits one or more major life activities. Cancer and its treatments, including chemotherapy, are generally considered disabilities under the ADA.

3. Reasonable Accommodations: Employers and educational institutions covered by the ADA are required to provide reasonable accommodations to individuals with disabilities. These accommodations are modifications or adjustments that enable individuals to perform essential job functions or participate in educational activities.

4. Interactive Process: The ADA mandates an interactive process between the individual and the employer or educational institution to determine

appropriate accommodations. This process involves open communication, sharing medical documentation, and exploring reasonable solutions.

Employment Protections:

Chemotherapy treatment may require individuals to navigate their work responsibilities while managing the physical and emotional challenges that accompany treatment. Several legal protections exist to support individuals in the workplace:

5. Family and Medical Leave Act (FMLA): FMLA provides eligible employees with up to 12 weeks of unpaid leave within a 12-month period for medical reasons, including cancer treatment. This allows individuals to take time off for chemotherapy without the risk of losing their job.

6. Workplace Accommodations: Under the ADA, employers are required to provide reasonable accommodations to individuals undergoing chemotherapy treatment. Accommodations may include flexible work hours, modified workstations, schedule adjustments, or temporary reassignment to less physically demanding tasks.

7. Disability Insurance: Short-term or long-term disability insurance coverage, often provided by employers, can offer income protection during periods of chemotherapy treatment. Individuals should review their insurance policies and understand the requirements and application process for disability benefits.

8. Anti-Discrimination Laws: Discrimination based on cancer diagnosis or chemotherapy treatment is prohibited under federal and state anti-discrimination laws. Employers cannot make hiring, firing, or promotional decisions based on an individual's medical condition or treatment.

Educational Accommodations:

Students facing chemotherapy treatment also have legal rights and protections in educational settings. These include:

9. Section 504 of the Rehabilitation Act: Section 504 prohibits discrimination against individuals with disabilities in federally-funded educational institutions. This includes providing reasonable accommodations to students facing chemotherapy treatment.

10. Individualized Education Program (IEP): If a student's chemotherapy treatment affects their ability to learn, they may be eligible for an IEP, which outlines individualized accommodations and support services tailored to their needs.

11. Homebound or Hospital Education: In cases where students are unable to attend school due to chemotherapy treatment, homebound or hospital education services may be provided. These services ensure that students continue their education and receive appropriate support during their treatment.

12. Communication with School Administration: It is essential for students and their families to communicate with school administrators about the need for accommodations, schedule adjustments, or modified coursework during chemotherapy treatment. Working together, families and educational professionals can develop appropriate plans to support the student's educational needs.

Requesting Accommodations:

When requesting accommodations, it is important to follow established procedures and provide the necessary documentation. Here are some steps to consider:

13. Documentation: Obtain medical documentation from healthcare providers detailing the diagnosis, treatment plan, and the need for specific accommodations.

Written Request

## Returning to work or school after treatment

Completing chemotherapy treatment is a significant milestone, but the journey doesn't end there. Individuals often face the challenge of transitioning back to work or school after chemotherapy. This period requires careful consideration of physical and emotional well-being, as well as effective communication and planning. This chapter explores the process of returning to work or school after chemotherapy, providing factual information and practical insights to empower individuals during this important phase.

Physical and Emotional Readiness:

Returning to work or school after chemotherapy requires considering one's physical and emotional readiness. It is crucial to assess whether sufficient healing and recovery have taken place. Consider the following factors:

2. Medical Clearance: Obtain medical clearance from healthcare providers before returning to work or school. This ensures that any physical restrictions or limitations are addressed and that the individual is deemed fit to resume regular activities.

3. Energy Levels: Chemotherapy treatment can cause fatigue, which may persist even after treatment ends. It's important to evaluate energy levels and determine whether they are sufficient to meet the demands of work or school.

4. Emotional Well-being: Chemotherapy can have emotional and psychological impacts. Evaluate emotional readiness and seek support from counselors, therapists, or support groups if needed.

Communicating with Employers or Educators:

Open and effective communication with employers or educators is essential when planning to return to work or school after chemotherapy. Consider the following strategies:

5. Informing about Treatment: Keep employers or educators informed about the chemotherapy treatment schedule and duration. Share updates on treatment completion and expected return dates.

6. Treatment Side Effects: Discuss any potential side effects that may impact work or school performance. Provide information on how these side effects can be managed and suggest accommodations if necessary.

7. Accommodation Requests: If required, request accommodations that will support a smooth transition back to work or school. This may include modified work hours, reduced workload, flexible scheduling, or adjustments to the learning environment.

Gradual Return and Flexible Arrangements:

Returning to full-time work or school immediately after chemotherapy may not be feasible. A gradual return or flexible arrangements can help ease the transition. Consider the following approaches:

8. Gradual Return: Begin with a part-time schedule or reduced hours and gradually increase workload over time. This allows individuals to assess their energy levels and adjust their pace accordingly.

9. Flexible Work or School Arrangements: Explore options for flexible work hours or remote work arrangements, if applicable. For students,

discuss with educators the possibility of modified schedules or remote learning options.

10. Modified Tasks: Request temporary modifications to work or school tasks or responsibilities to accommodate any lingering physical limitations or side effects. Collaborate with employers or educators to identify reasonable adjustments.

Building Support Networks:

Returning to work or school after chemotherapy can be emotionally challenging. Building a support network provides a sense of belonging and assistance during this transition period. Consider the following strategies:

11. Colleague or Classmate Support: Share experiences and concerns with understanding colleagues or classmates who can provide support and empathy.

12. Employee Assistance Programs (EAP): Utilize any EAP services offered by employers to access counseling, mental health support, or other resources.

13. Support Groups: Engage with cancer survivor support groups or online communities where individuals share similar experiences and can provide advice and encouragement.

Self-Care and Work-Life Balance:

Maintaining self-care practices and a healthy work-life balance is crucial when returning to work or school after chemotherapy. Consider the following approaches:

14. Prioritize Self-Care: Continue practicing self-care routines established during chemotherapy, such as getting adequate sleep, eating a balanced diet, and engaging in stress-relieving activities.

15. Set Boundaries: Establish clear boundaries between work or school and personal life to prevent burnout. Allocate time for hobbies, relaxation, and spending quality time with

Chapter Twelve

# Chemotherapy in Children and Adolescents

When it comes to cancer treatment, chemotherapy plays a crucial role in the care of children and adolescents. Although facing a cancer diagnosis at a young age is challenging, advances in medical technology and treatment options have significantly improved outcomes. This chapter explores the use of chemotherapy in children and adolescents, providing factual information and insights into the unique considerations and approaches to ensure the best possible outcomes for these young patients.

Importance of Chemotherapy in Pediatric Oncology:

Chemotherapy is a key component of cancer treatment in children and adolescents. It involves the use of powerful medications to target and kill cancer cells. Chemotherapy may be used as a standalone treatment or in combination with other modalities, such as surgery or radiation therapy. The goals of chemotherapy in pediatric oncology include:

2. Shrinkage or elimination of tumors: Chemotherapy aims to reduce the size of tumors or eradicate them entirely, improving the chances of long-term remission or cure.

3. Preventing the spread of cancer: Chemotherapy can help prevent cancer cells from spreading to other parts of the body, reducing the risk of metastasis.

4. Treating leukemia and lymphomas: Chemotherapy is a primary treatment for leukemia and lymphomas, which are the most common types of cancer in children.

Special Considerations for Pediatric Chemotherapy:

Chemotherapy in children and adolescents requires special considerations due to their unique physiological and psychological characteristics. Understanding these considerations helps healthcare professionals tailor treatment plans and provide optimal care:

5. Dose Adjustments: Children may require dose adjustments based on factors such as body weight, age, and individual tolerance. Medications are often calculated based on body surface area to ensure safe and effective treatment.

6. Growth and Development: Chemotherapy can affect a child's growth and development. Close monitoring is necessary to detect any developmental delays or growth abnormalities early and provide appropriate interventions.

7. Fertility Preservation: Some chemotherapy drugs can have long-term effects on fertility. Discussing fertility preservation options with the healthcare team before treatment is important for adolescents who may want to have children in the future.

8. Emotional Support: Children and adolescents undergoing chemotherapy require specialized emotional support. This may involve the involvement of child life specialists, psychologists, or social workers to help children understand and cope with their treatment.

Chemotherapy Administration:

Chemotherapy can be administered in various ways to children and adolescents, depending on the specific cancer type and treatment plan:

9. Intravenous (IV) Infusion: IV infusion is the most common method of administering chemotherapy in pediatric patients. Medications are delivered directly into a vein using a needle or a central venous access device (CVAD).

10. Oral Medications: Some chemotherapy drugs can be taken orally, in the form of pills or liquid. This method provides convenience for children and allows for treatment to be administered at home.

11. Intrathecal Chemotherapy: For certain types of cancer, chemotherapy may need to be delivered directly into the cerebrospinal fluid. This is done through a procedure called intrathecal chemotherapy, which involves the injection of medications into the spinal canal.

12. Targeted Therapies: In addition to traditional chemotherapy, targeted therapies are increasingly used in pediatric oncology. These medications specifically target cancer cells while minimizing damage to healthy cells, thereby reducing side effects.

Managing Side Effects:

Chemotherapy can cause side effects in children and adolescents, impacting their quality of life. It is important to manage these side effects effectively to ensure the well-being of young patients:

13. Nausea and Vomiting: Anti-nausea medications may be prescribed to minimize nausea and vomiting associated with chemotherapy. Encouraging small, frequent meals and providing comfort measures can also help alleviate these symptoms.

14. Hair Loss: Hair loss is a common side effect of certain chemotherapy drugs.

## Unique considerations for young patients

When it comes to chemotherapy treatment, young patients have specific needs and considerations that require specialized care and attention. Children and adolescents undergoing chemotherapy face unique challenges related to their physical and emotional development. This chapter explores the unique considerations for young patients undergoing chemotherapy, providing factual information and insights into the importance of tailored care for this vulnerable population.

Physiological Considerations:

Young patients undergoing chemotherapy have unique physiological considerations that influence treatment decisions and management. Understanding these factors helps healthcare providers deliver personalized care:

2. Age-Related Differences: Children and adolescents have distinct physiological characteristics compared to adults. Their bodies are still developing, and organ systems may have different tolerances and responses to chemotherapy drugs.

3. Growth and Development: Chemotherapy treatment during childhood and adolescence can impact growth and development. Certain chemotherapy drugs may affect bone development, hormonal balance, or reproductive functions. Regular monitoring and interventions are necessary to ensure optimal growth and development.

4. Dose Adjustments: Chemotherapy doses for young patients are typically calculated based on body surface area or weight to ensure appropriate

dosing. These calculations consider the child's age, size, and individual tolerance to minimize toxicity and optimize treatment outcomes.

Emotional and Psychological Considerations:

Young patients undergoing chemotherapy face emotional and psychological challenges that require special attention and support. Addressing these considerations is vital for their overall well-being:

5. Age-Appropriate Communication: Healthcare providers need to communicate with young patients using age-appropriate language and explanations. Ensuring that children understand their diagnosis, treatment plan, and potential side effects can reduce anxiety and foster active participation in their care.

6. Psychosocial Support: Emotional support is crucial for young patients undergoing chemotherapy. Child life specialists, psychologists, and social workers play important roles in providing psychosocial support, helping children cope with treatment-related stress, and addressing any concerns or fears they may have.

7. School and Social Integration: Chemotherapy treatment can disrupt a child's academic and social life. School reintegration programs and support services can help young patients continue their education, maintain social connections, and adjust to changes caused by treatment.

Family Involvement and Support:

The involvement of families is paramount when caring for young patients undergoing chemotherapy. The family plays a crucial role in providing emotional support and facilitating the child's well-being:

8. Caregiver Education: Educating parents or caregivers about the chemotherapy treatment plan, potential side effects, and ways to support

their child is essential. This includes instructions on managing medications, recognizing and responding to side effects, and maintaining a safe and nurturing environment at home.

9. Sibling Support: Siblings of young patients also require attention and support. Their daily routines may be disrupted, and they may experience emotional challenges. Providing information and resources to siblings can help them understand and cope with their sibling's chemotherapy treatment.

10. Family-Centered Care: Family-centered care involves collaborative decision-making between healthcare providers and families, taking into account the unique needs and preferences of each patient and their family. It fosters a supportive and empowering environment that recognizes the family's expertise in their child's care.

Pediatric-Specific Support Services:

Pediatric oncology centers provide specialized support services to address the unique needs of young patients undergoing chemotherapy:

11. Play Therapy: Play therapy offers a therapeutic outlet for children, allowing them to express their emotions, fears, and concerns through play. It promotes psychological healing and coping skills development.

12. Art and Music Therapy: Art and music therapy provide creative outlets for self-expression and emotional healing. These therapies can enhance communication, reduce anxiety, and improve overall well-being for young patients.

13. School Programs: Pediatric oncology centers often have dedicated school programs or liaisons who work with the child's school to provide educational support and ensure a smooth transition back to the classroom.

## Emotional support for children and families

When children undergo chemotherapy, they face a unique set of emotional challenges that can impact their well-being and overall treatment experience. Additionally, the emotional well-being of their families plays a crucial role in providing a nurturing and supportive environment. This chapter explores the importance of emotional support for children and families during chemotherapy, offering factual information and practical insights into fostering resilience and well-being throughout the treatment journey.

Understanding the Emotional Impact:

Chemotherapy treatment can be overwhelming for children and their families. It is essential to recognize the emotional impact and address the following aspects:

2. Fear and Anxiety: Children may experience fear and anxiety related to the unfamiliarity of the treatment process, potential side effects, and disruption to their daily lives. Understanding their concerns and providing reassurance can help alleviate anxiety.

3. Sadness and Loss: Children may grieve the loss of their normal routines, school activities, and social interactions during treatment. Acknowledging their feelings of sadness and loss while providing opportunities for engagement and connection can support emotional well-being.

4. Uncertainty and Control: The unpredictable nature of chemotherapy can leave children feeling a lack of control over their bodies and lives. Empowering them with age-appropriate information and involving them in decision-making when possible can help restore a sense of control.

Child Life Specialists:

Child life specialists are integral members of the pediatric oncology team who specialize in supporting children and families throughout the treatment process. They focus on promoting emotional well-being and providing age-appropriate support:

5. Preparation for Procedures: Child life specialists use play and interactive techniques to prepare children for medical procedures, reducing anxiety and increasing understanding.

6. Emotional Expression: These specialists create safe spaces for children to express their feelings and concerns through play, art, or storytelling. They help children develop coping strategies and provide them with tools to navigate difficult emotions.

7. Sibling Support: Child life specialists also offer support to siblings of children undergoing chemotherapy. They provide age-appropriate explanations and engage siblings in therapeutic activities to help them understand and cope with their sibling's treatment.

Parent and Caregiver Support:

Parents and caregivers play a vital role in providing emotional support to their children during chemotherapy. It is essential to focus on their well-being as well:

8. Information and Education: Parents and caregivers benefit from receiving comprehensive information about the treatment plan, potential side effects, and available support services. This knowledge empowers them to better support their child and navigate the treatment journey.

9. Peer Support: Connecting parents and caregivers with support groups or online communities allows them to share experiences, exchange coping strategies, and find solace in knowing they are not alone. Peer support provides a valuable platform for emotional validation and resource sharing.

10. Self-Care Practices: Encouraging parents and caregivers to prioritize self-care is crucial for their own emotional well-being. Engaging in activities that promote relaxation, seeking support from friends and family, and seeking professional counseling when needed can help maintain their resilience.

Psychosocial Support Services:

Psychosocial support services within pediatric oncology centers offer a range of resources to address the emotional needs of children and families:

11. Individual and Family Counseling: Professional counseling services provide a safe and supportive environment for children and families to explore their emotions, address concerns, and develop coping strategies.

12. Support Groups: Joining support groups tailored for children or families allows them to connect with others going through similar experiences. These groups foster a sense of community, provide emotional validation, and offer opportunities for peer support.

13. Therapeutic Play and Expressive Arts: Art and play therapy provide avenues for children to express their feelings, fears, and hopes in a non-verbal and creative way. These therapies facilitate emotional healing and serve as tools for communication and self-expression.

Integration of School and Social

## Long-term effects and follow-up care

Chemotherapy is a cornerstone of cancer treatment, but its effects extend beyond the immediate treatment period. Long-term effects may arise months or even years after completion of chemotherapy, warranting ongoing follow-up care. This chapter explores the long-term effects of chemotherapy and the importance of comprehensive follow-up care, providing factual information and insights into promoting the health and well-being of individuals who have undergone chemotherapy.

Late Effects of Chemotherapy:

Chemotherapy can have various long-term effects on the body, even after treatment has ended. These effects may vary depending on factors such as the type of cancer, specific chemotherapy drugs used, dosage, and individual susceptibility. Some common long-term effects include:

2. Cardiac Issues: Certain chemotherapy drugs may damage the heart, leading to long-term cardiovascular problems. Regular cardiac monitoring and preventive measures, such as lifestyle modifications, may be recommended.

3. Cognitive Changes: Chemotherapy-related cognitive changes, often referred to as "chemo brain," can manifest as memory problems, difficulty concentrating, and decreased mental processing speed. Rehabilitation programs and cognitive exercises can help manage these changes.

4. Endocrine Dysfunction: Chemotherapy may affect hormone production and regulation, resulting in endocrine-related issues such as thyroid dysfunction, growth hormone deficiency, or reproductive system impairment. Regular endocrine monitoring and hormone replacement therapy, if necessary, can address these concerns.

5. Secondary Cancers: Some chemotherapy drugs may increase the risk of developing secondary cancers later in life. Regular screenings and ongoing surveillance are crucial to detect and manage any potential malignancies.

6. Emotional and Psychological Well-being: The emotional and psychological impact of chemotherapy can persist beyond treatment. Individuals may experience anxiety, depression, or post-traumatic stress disorder.

Ongoing psychological support and counseling can aid in managing these long-term effects.

Importance of Follow-Up Care:

Comprehensive follow-up care is essential to monitor and address potential long-term effects of chemotherapy. Regular medical check-ups, screenings, and consultations with healthcare providers play a vital role in ensuring optimal health and well-being. Key aspects of follow-up care include:

7. Medical Monitoring: Regular medical check-ups allow healthcare providers to monitor the individual's overall health, address any emerging concerns, and identify potential late effects of chemotherapy. This may involve physical examinations, blood tests, imaging studies, and other specialized assessments.

8. Surveillance for Secondary Cancers: Due to the increased risk of secondary cancers, ongoing surveillance is crucial. Screening tests, such as mammograms, colonoscopies, or skin examinations, may be recommended based on the individual's specific treatment history and risk factors.

9. Psychological Support: Emotional and psychological well-being should be an integral part of follow-up care. Ongoing counseling, support groups, or referral to mental health professionals can provide individuals with the tools to cope with any psychological challenges that may arise.

10. Lifestyle Recommendations: Encouraging a healthy lifestyle is essential for individuals who have undergone chemotherapy. Recommendations may include maintaining a balanced diet, engaging in regular physical activity, managing stress, and avoiding tobacco and excessive alcohol consumption.

Survivorship Care Plans:

Survivorship care plans are comprehensive documents that outline the individual's cancer treatment history, potential long-term effects, and recommended follow-up care. These plans provide a roadmap for healthcare providers, patients, and caregivers to ensure coordinated and personalized care. Key components of survivorship care plans include:

11. Treatment Summary: A summary of the individual's specific chemotherapy treatment, including the drugs used, dosage, duration, and any other relevant details.

12. Long-Term Follow-Up Guidelines: Detailed guidelines outlining recommended follow-up care, including screenings, tests, and consultations with various healthcare providers.

13. Potential Late Effects: Information on potential long-term effects of chemotherapy, empowering individuals to recognize symptoms and seek appropriate medical attention.

Lifestyle Recommendations

Chapter Thirteen

# Chemotherapy for Older Adults

As the population ages, an increasing number of older adults are diagnosed with cancer and undergo chemotherapy treatment. While chemotherapy can be an effective option for older adults, this age group often faces unique considerations that must be taken into account to ensure personalized and effective care. This chapter explores the use of chemotherapy in older adults, providing factual information and insights into the importance of tailored treatment approaches for this population.

Considerations in Older Adults:

Older adults undergoing chemotherapy require specialized care due to various factors that may influence treatment decisions and outcomes:

2. Age-Related Changes: Aging affects the body's physiology, including decreased organ function and changes in metabolism. These factors can impact the body's ability to tolerate and process chemotherapy drugs.

3. Existing Health Conditions: Older adults may have pre-existing health conditions, such as heart disease, diabetes, or kidney impairment. These conditions may influence treatment decisions, drug choices, and dosage adjustments.

4. Polypharmacy: Older adults often take multiple medications for chronic conditions. Interactions between chemotherapy drugs and other medications must be carefully considered to prevent adverse effects or reduced treatment efficacy.

5. Functional Status: Assessing an older adult's functional status is crucial to determine their ability to tolerate chemotherapy and manage potential side effects. Factors such as mobility, cognition, and social support play a role in treatment decision-making.

Individualized Treatment Decisions:

Chemotherapy treatment decisions for older adults should be individualized, taking into account the specific characteristics and needs of each patient:

6. Comprehensive Geriatric Assessment (CGA): A CGA is a comprehensive evaluation that assesses an older adult's overall health, functional status, psychological well-being, and social support. This assessment helps guide treatment decisions and identify potential vulnerabilities.

7. Treatment Goals: The goals of chemotherapy may vary for older adults. Some may prioritize extending survival, while others may focus on maintaining quality of life and functional independence. Open and honest communication between healthcare providers and patients is essential in determining treatment goals.

8. Drug Selection and Dosage: Certain chemotherapy drugs may be better suited for older adults due to their tolerability and safety profiles. Dosage adjustments may be necessary based on factors such as renal function and overall health status.

9. Comorbidity Management: Managing pre-existing health conditions is crucial in older adults. Close coordination between oncologists and other specialists is necessary to optimize overall health and ensure that chemotherapy treatment is safely integrated into the individual's care plan.

Managing Side Effects:

Chemotherapy side effects can be particularly challenging for older adults. Strategies to manage side effects should be tailored to their specific needs:

10. Toxicity and Tolerance: Older adults may be more vulnerable to chemotherapy-related toxicity due to age-related changes in organ function. Close monitoring of treatment response and potential side effects is essential to make timely adjustments and optimize tolerability.

11. Supportive Care: Supportive care interventions, such as antiemetics for nausea and vomiting, growth factors to reduce the risk of infection, or blood transfusions for anemia, can be incorporated to mitigate side effects and improve quality of life during chemotherapy.

12. Geriatric Oncology Specialists: Collaboration with geriatric oncology specialists can provide valuable expertise in managing side effects and optimizing treatment outcomes for older adults.

Comprehensive Geriatric Support:

Older adults undergoing chemotherapy benefit from comprehensive geriatric support services to address their unique needs:

13. Geriatric Oncology Clinics: Geriatric oncology clinics specialize in providing multidisciplinary care tailored to older adults. These clinics often incorporate geriatricians, oncologists, nurses, and other healthcare professionals with expertise in the care of older cancer patients.

14. Functional Assessment and Rehabilitation: Rehabilitation services, such as physical therapy, occupational therapy, and speech therapy, can help older adults maintain or regain functional independence during and after chemotherapy.

## Age-related factors in treatment

Age plays a significant role in how individuals respond to chemotherapy treatment. Various age-related factors can influence treatment decisions, response rates, and the overall management of side effects. Understanding these factors is crucial for healthcare professionals to provide personalized and effective care. This chapter explores age-related factors in chemotherapy treatment, highlighting the importance of tailoring care to different age groups.

Younger Adults:

Younger adults, typically defined as individuals between the ages of 18 and 39, often have unique considerations when it comes to chemotherapy treatment:

2. Physical Resilience: Younger adults generally have better physical reserves and tolerate chemotherapy more effectively than older age groups. This allows for the administration of more aggressive treatment regimens.

3. Fertility Preservation: Chemotherapy can have a significant impact on fertility. Younger adults who desire to have children may opt for fertility preservation methods before starting chemotherapy, such as sperm or egg freezing.

4. Long-Term Survivorship: With longer life expectancies, younger adults are more likely to face long-term survivorship challenges after chemotherapy treatment. These challenges include monitoring for late effects, managing potential secondary cancers, and addressing psychological and emotional concerns.

Older Adults:

Older adults, typically defined as individuals aged 65 and older, present unique considerations in chemotherapy treatment due to the physiological and psychosocial changes associated with aging:

5. Physiological Changes: Aging is associated with physiological changes that may affect the pharmacokinetics and pharmacodynamics of chemotherapy drugs. These changes can influence drug metabolism, drug clearance, and drug toxicity.

6. Comorbidities: Older adults often have multiple comorbidities, such as cardiovascular disease, diabetes, or kidney dysfunction. These conditions may impact treatment decisions, drug selection, and dosage adjustments to minimize the risk of adverse events.

7. Functional Status: Assessing an older adult's functional status is crucial for determining their ability to tolerate chemotherapy treatment. Factors such as mobility, cognitive function, and social support play a role in treatment decision-making.

8. Polypharmacy: Older adults commonly take multiple medications for chronic conditions. It is essential to evaluate potential drug interactions and adjust treatment plans accordingly to prevent adverse drug reactions or reduced treatment efficacy.

9. Geriatric Syndromes: Older adults may experience geriatric syndromes such as falls, cognitive impairment, or frailty. These syndromes can impact treatment decisions and require additional management and support during chemotherapy.

Pediatric and Adolescent Patients:

Chemotherapy treatment in pediatric and adolescent patients requires specialized care due to their unique physiological and psychosocial characteristics:

10. Physiological Considerations: Children and adolescents have distinct physiological characteristics compared to adults. Their bodies are still developing, and organ systems may have different tolerances and responses

to chemotherapy drugs. Dose adjustments are often based on factors such as body surface area and weight.

11. Emotional and Psychological Support: Children and adolescents undergoing chemotherapy require age-appropriate emotional and psychological support. Child life specialists, psychologists, and social workers play vital roles in providing psychosocial support and addressing their specific needs.

12. School and Social Integration: Chemotherapy treatment can disrupt a child's academic and social life. School reintegration programs and support services are crucial to ensure continuity of education, maintain social connections, and support the emotional well-being of pediatric and adolescent patients.

Cultural Considerations:

Cultural factors can significantly influence how individuals perceive and approach chemotherapy treatment:

13. Beliefs and Values: Cultural beliefs and values surrounding health and illness may impact treatment decisions and adherence. Understanding and respecting these beliefs is essential for effective communication and shared decision-making.

14. Language and Communication: Language barriers can hinder effective communication between healthcare providers and patients. Access to interpreters or culturally competent healthcare professionals can help overcome these challenges and ensure clear understanding of treatment plans available.

## Managing multiple health conditions

When individuals undergo chemotherapy, managing multiple health conditions can present unique challenges. Coexisting medical conditions, such as diabetes, cardiovascular disease, or autoimmune disorders, require careful consideration and coordination to ensure safe and effective chemotherapy treatment. This chapter explores the importance of managing multiple health conditions during chemotherapy, providing factual information and insights into navigating the complexities of treatment in individuals with preexisting medical conditions.

Comprehensive Assessment:

Comprehensive assessment of an individual's medical history, including preexisting conditions, is vital in the management of chemotherapy treatment. The following factors should be considered:

2. Medical History: A thorough review of the individual's medical history helps identify coexisting conditions, their severity, and their potential impact on chemotherapy treatment. It allows healthcare providers to develop personalized treatment plans and make appropriate adjustments.

3. Medication Review: An assessment of the individual's medication regimen is necessary to identify potential drug interactions or contraindications with chemotherapy drugs. Collaboration between the oncology team and specialists managing other conditions is crucial in optimizing medication management.

4. Baseline Evaluations: Baseline evaluations of organ function, such as cardiac, renal, or liver function tests, help establish a foundation for monitoring potential chemotherapy-related toxicities and guide treatment decisions.

Multidisciplinary Approach:

Managing multiple health conditions during chemotherapy requires a collaborative, multidisciplinary approach involving healthcare providers from different specialties:

5. Oncology Team: The oncology team, consisting of medical oncologists, nurses, and pharmacists, plays a central role in managing chemotherapy treatment. They collaborate with other specialists to develop a comprehensive treatment plan that accounts for coexisting conditions.

6. Specialists: Specialists managing preexisting conditions, such as cardiologists, endocrinologists, or rheumatologists, contribute their expertise in assessing and managing the individual's specific health needs. They work closely with the oncology team to ensure coordinated care and optimize treatment outcomes.

7. Primary Care Providers: Primary care providers play an important role in coordinating care among various specialists, monitoring overall health, and addressing general health concerns outside the realm of chemotherapy treatment.

Individualized Treatment Planning:

Individualized treatment planning is crucial when managing multiple health conditions during chemotherapy. Considerations include:

8. Chemotherapy Drug Selection: The choice of chemotherapy drugs takes into account their potential impact on preexisting conditions. Some drugs may be better tolerated or have fewer interactions with specific conditions, guiding treatment decisions.

9. Dosage Adjustments: Dosage adjustments may be necessary to minimize the risk of toxicity or adverse events in individuals with preexisting conditions. Adjustments ensure that chemotherapy remains safe and effective while considering the individual's overall health status.

10. Treatment Sequence: The sequence in which chemotherapy and other treatments are administered may be modified to accommodate preexisting conditions. This sequencing optimizes the individual's overall health and minimizes potential interactions.

Close Monitoring and Communication:

Close monitoring and ongoing communication among healthcare providers are essential to ensure the safe management of multiple health conditions during chemotherapy:

11. Regular Follow-up: Regular follow-up appointments with the oncology team and other specialists involved in the individual's care help monitor treatment response, assess side effects, and address any emerging concerns or complications.

12. Open Communication: Effective communication among healthcare providers, the individual, and their support system is vital. This promotes coordination of care, enables timely interventions, and ensures that all parties are aware of the individual's specific needs and treatment plan.

13. Symptom Management: Proactive symptom management is crucial in individuals with multiple health conditions. Prompt identification and treatment of chemotherapy-related side effects help mitigate the impact on preexisting conditions and overall well-being.

Patient Empowerment:

Empowering individuals to actively participate in their care is key to managing multiple health conditions during chemotherapy:

14. Education and Information: Providing comprehensive education

## Caregiving and support for older patients

When older patients undergo chemotherapy, they often rely on the support and care provided by their loved ones or caregivers. The role of caregivers is crucial in ensuring the well-being and comfort of older patients throughout their chemotherapy journey. This chapter explores the importance of caregiving and support for older patients undergoing chemotherapy, offering factual information and insights into how caregivers can provide effective care and support during this challenging time.

Understanding the Caregiver's Role:

Caregivers play a vital role in the care and support of older patients undergoing chemotherapy. Understanding their responsibilities and challenges is essential for effective caregiving:

2. Emotional Support: Caregivers provide emotional support by offering comfort, reassurance, and empathy to older patients. They create a safe and nurturing environment that helps alleviate anxiety and promotes a positive mindset.

3. Practical Assistance: Caregivers assist with practical tasks such as scheduling medical appointments, managing medications, providing transportation, and coordinating communication with healthcare providers.

4. Advocacy: Caregivers advocate for the needs and preferences of older patients, ensuring that their voices are heard and their choices respected throughout the chemotherapy process.

5. Information and Education: Caregivers seek and share information about chemotherapy treatment, potential side effects, and available support resources. They help older patients understand their treatment plans and make informed decisions.

Physical Care and Comfort:

Physical care and comfort are vital aspects of caregiving for older patients undergoing chemotherapy. Caregivers can provide support in the following ways:

6. Personal Care Assistance: Caregivers help older patients with activities of daily living, such as bathing, dressing, grooming, and maintaining oral hygiene. They ensure the patient's physical well-being and comfort.

7. Nutrition and Hydration: Caregivers assist with meal planning and preparation to ensure that older patients receive proper nutrition during chemotherapy. They encourage hydration and monitor any dietary restrictions or preferences.

8. Medication Management: Caregivers help older patients adhere to their medication schedules, ensuring that chemotherapy drugs and other medications are taken as prescribed. They also monitor for any potential drug interactions or side effects.

9. Pain Management: Caregivers play a crucial role in monitoring and managing pain experienced by older patients during chemotherapy. They work closely with healthcare providers to ensure appropriate pain management strategies are in place.

Providing Emotional Support:

Emotional support is essential for the well-being of older patients undergoing chemotherapy. Caregivers can provide the following forms of emotional support:

10. Active Listening: Caregivers listen attentively to the concerns, fears, and emotions expressed by older patients. They create a safe space for open communication and provide a supportive presence.

11. Encouragement and Motivation: Caregivers offer words of encouragement and motivation to uplift the spirits of older patients during challenging times. They help foster a positive mindset and promote resilience.

12. Engagement in Meaningful Activities: Caregivers facilitate engagement in activities that bring joy and meaning to older patients' lives. This may include hobbies, social interactions, or participation in support groups.

13. Psychological Support: Caregivers recognize and address any signs of anxiety, depression, or emotional distress in older patients. They encourage seeking professional support, such as counseling or therapy, when needed.

Practical Considerations:

Caregiving for older patients undergoing chemotherapy involves practical considerations to ensure a safe and comfortable environment:

14. Safety Precautions: Caregivers assess the home environment to identify and address any potential safety hazards. They ensure that the living space is free from obstacles, well-lit, and equipped with necessary assistive devices if needed.

15. Transportation and Accompaniment: Caregivers arrange transportation to and from medical appointments, chemotherapy sessions, and other healthcare-related visits. They provide companionship and support during these visits.

Communication with Healthcare

## Clinical Trials and Emerging Treatments

Chapter Fourteen

# Chemotherapy has long been a cornerstone of cancer treatment, but the field continues to evolve with ongoing clinical trials and the emergence of new treatment approaches. Clinical trials play a vital role in advancing chemotherapy and improving patient outcomes. This chapter explores the significance of clinical trials and emerging treatments in relation to chemotherapy, providing factual information

# and insights into their impact on the future of cancer care.

2. Clinical Trials: Advancing Scientific Knowledge

Clinical trials are research studies designed to evaluate the safety and effectiveness of new treatments, including chemotherapy regimens. They aim to advance scientific knowledge and improve patient care in several ways:

3. Treatment Efficacy: Clinical trials assess the effectiveness of new chemotherapy treatments by comparing them to standard treatments or alternative approaches. These trials provide evidence on the benefits and potential risks of novel therapies.

4. Treatment Personalization: Clinical trials help identify patient populations that are more likely to respond favorably to specific chemotherapy regimens. This knowledge aids in tailoring treatment decisions based on individual characteristics, improving outcomes and reducing unnecessary side effects.

5. New Drug Development: Clinical trials test new chemotherapy drugs or drug combinations to expand the available treatment options. This research fosters innovation and the discovery of more effective and targeted therapies.

6. Treatment Optimization: Clinical trials explore ways to optimize chemotherapy treatment by assessing different dosages, treatment sched-

ules, and combinations. This knowledge helps refine treatment protocols and maximize therapeutic benefits.

Phases of Clinical Trials:

Clinical trials follow a systematic process consisting of several phases:

7. Phase 1: Phase 1 trials evaluate the safety and dosage of a new chemotherapy drug in a small group of patients. The focus is on determining the maximum tolerated dose and identifying potential side effects.

8. Phase 2: Phase 2 trials involve a larger group of patients and assess the effectiveness of the new chemotherapy treatment. Researchers gather more data on the drug's efficacy, safety, and optimal dosage.

9. Phase 3: Phase 3 trials compare the new chemotherapy treatment to the standard treatment in a large group of patients. These trials provide more robust evidence on treatment efficacy, safety, and potential benefits over existing therapies.

10. Phase 4: Phase 4 trials, also known as post-marketing trials, occur after a treatment is approved for clinical use. These trials monitor the long-term effects, safety, and effectiveness of the chemotherapy treatment in a larger population.

Targeted Therapies and Immunotherapy:

Emerging treatments in the field of chemotherapy include targeted therapies and immunotherapy, which offer new approaches to cancer treatment:

11. Targeted Therapies: Targeted therapies are designed to specifically attack cancer cells by targeting specific molecules or pathways involved in tumor growth. Unlike traditional chemotherapy, which affects both

healthy and cancerous cells, targeted therapies aim to minimize damage to healthy cells, reducing side effects.

12. Immunotherapy: Immunotherapy harnesses the body's immune system to fight cancer cells. It stimulates or enhances the immune response to identify and destroy cancer cells. Immunotherapies can be used alone or in combination with chemotherapy to improve treatment outcomes.

Personalized Medicine:

Advancements in genomic research have paved the way for personalized medicine, tailoring treatment to an individual's specific genetic makeup:

13. Biomarker Testing: Biomarker testing analyzes specific genetic or molecular characteristics of a tumor to identify biomarkers that can guide treatment decisions. This testing helps determine if a patient is likely to respond to a particular chemotherapy treatment.

14. Precision Medicine: Precision medicine utilizes biomarker testing and genetic profiling to select the most effective chemotherapy treatment for each patient. It aims to optimize treatment outcomes by targeting the specific genetic alterations driving the cancer.

Collaboration and Knowledge Sharing:

Collaboration and knowledge sharing are vital in advancing chemotherapy treatment through clinical trials and emerging therapies:

Multid

## Understanding clinical trials

Clinical trials are at the forefront of medical research, playing a critical role in advancing chemotherapy treatments and improving patient outcomes.

These trials are designed to rigorously test new interventions, including chemotherapy regimens, and provide valuable insights into their safety, effectiveness, and potential benefits. This chapter aims to demystify the world of clinical trials, shedding light on their significance in the context of chemotherapy and providing factual information to foster a better understanding.

The Purpose of Clinical Trials:

Clinical trials serve several important purposes, including:

2. Assessing Safety: Clinical trials evaluate the safety of new chemotherapy treatments by carefully monitoring patients for adverse effects, complications, or unexpected reactions. This ensures that potential risks are identified and mitigated.

3. Determining Efficacy: Clinical trials aim to determine the effectiveness of new chemotherapy regimens compared to existing standard treatments or alternative approaches. They provide evidence on the potential benefits and outcomes associated with novel interventions.

4. Tailoring Treatment: Clinical trials help identify patient populations that are more likely to respond favorably to specific chemotherapy regimens. This knowledge aids in tailoring treatment decisions based on individual characteristics, improving treatment outcomes and reducing unnecessary side effects.

5. Expanding Treatment Options: Clinical trials play a pivotal role in expanding the range of available chemotherapy treatments. They test new drugs, drug combinations, dosages, and treatment schedules, opening doors to more effective and targeted therapies.

The Phases of Clinical Trials:

Clinical trials follow a systematic progression through various phases:

6. Phase 1: Phase 1 trials involve a small group of patients and primarily focus on evaluating the safety and dosage of a new chemotherapy drug. Researchers aim to determine the maximum tolerated dose and identify any potential side effects.

7. Phase 2: Phase 2 trials expand the participant pool and assess the efficacy of the new chemotherapy treatment. These trials gather more data on the drug's effectiveness, safety, and optimal dosage, often involving patients with specific cancer types.

8. Phase 3: Phase 3 trials involve a larger population of patients and compare the new chemotherapy treatment to the standard treatment. These trials provide robust evidence on treatment efficacy, safety, and potential benefits over existing therapies.

9. Phase 4: Phase 4 trials, also known as post-marketing trials, occur after a treatment has received regulatory approval. They monitor the long-term effects, safety, and effectiveness of the chemotherapy treatment in a larger population.

Ethical Considerations and Patient Safety:

Clinical trials adhere to strict ethical guidelines and prioritize patient safety:

10. Informed Consent: Prior to participation, individuals are provided with comprehensive information about the trial, including its purpose, potential risks and benefits, and the procedures involved. Informed consent ensures that participants understand and voluntarily agree to participate.

11. Institutional Review Boards (IRBs): Clinical trials undergo rigorous ethical review by IRBs, which assess the trial's scientific validity, safety measures, and potential benefits. IRBs aim to protect the rights and welfare of trial participants.

12. Monitoring and Oversight: Clinical trials are closely monitored by dedicated teams, including researchers, clinicians, and independent monitors. They ensure compliance with protocols, monitor patient safety, and analyze trial data.

Collaboration and Knowledge Sharing:

Collaboration and knowledge sharing are key components of successful clinical trials:

13. Multidisciplinary Teams: Clinical trials involve collaboration among diverse healthcare professionals, including researchers, oncologists, nurses, pharmacists, and statisticians. Their collective expertise ensures comprehensive and accurate data collection and analysis.

14. Data Sharing and Analysis: Clinical trial data is often shared among researchers and institutions, facilitating collaboration and further analysis. This data sharing helps advance scientific knowledge and encourages innovation in chemotherapy treatment.

Benefits and Risks of Participation:

Participating in a clinical trial can have both benefits

## Eligibility and participation

Clinical trials are vital in advancing chemotherapy treatments and improving patient outcomes. However, not everyone is eligible to participate in these trials, and careful consideration must be given to ensure the safety and effectiveness of the interventions being tested. This chapter explores the factors that determine eligibility and the considerations individuals must take into account when deciding to participate in clinical trials related to chemotherapy. By understanding the criteria and processes involved, individuals can make informed decisions about their potential involvement in these groundbreaking studies.

Eligibility Criteria:

Clinical trials have specific eligibility criteria that must be met to ensure the suitability of participants. The criteria vary depending on the trial's objectives, the specific chemotherapy treatment being studied, and the type of cancer being targeted. Some common eligibility factors include:

2. Cancer Type and Stage: Clinical trials often focus on specific types and stages of cancer. Eligibility may be restricted to patients with a particular diagnosis or cancer subtype, as this helps researchers gather more precise data on the treatment's efficacy for that specific condition.

3. Age and Gender: Some clinical trials may have age or gender restrictions, especially if the treatment is being tested in specific populations, such as pediatric or elderly patients, or if the intervention targets certain biological differences.

4. Medical History and Health Status: Participants' medical history and overall health play a crucial role in eligibility. Certain preexisting medical conditions or comorbidities may disqualify individuals due to potential interactions or risks associated with the experimental treatment.

5. Prior Treatments: The availability of previous treatments and the individual's response to those treatments are important factors. Some trials may exclude patients who have already received specific chemotherapy regimens or other therapies that could affect the trial's results.

6. Performance Status: Performance status measures a patient's overall functional ability and well-being. Trials may require participants to meet specific performance status criteria to ensure they can tolerate the study procedures and follow-up assessments.

Informed Consent and Decision-Making:

Participating in a clinical trial is a voluntary decision that requires informed consent. Several considerations should be taken into account when deciding to participate:

7. Informed Consent Process: Individuals considering participation in a clinical trial receive comprehensive information about the trial, including its purpose, procedures, potential risks and benefits, and alternatives. They have the opportunity to ask questions and fully understand what their involvement entails before providing informed consent.

8. Benefits and Risks: Understanding the potential benefits and risks of participation is crucial. Clinical trials offer the possibility of accessing innovative treatments, receiving close monitoring and follow-up care, and contributing to medical knowledge. However, there may also be unknown risks associated with the experimental treatment or additional procedures involved.

9. Alternative Treatment Options: It is important to discuss alternative treatment options with healthcare providers before making a decision. Comparing the potential benefits of the clinical trial with standard treatments is crucial in determining the best course of action for individual cases.

10. Right to Withdraw: Individuals have the right to withdraw from a clinical trial at any time, without jeopardizing their future care or treatment options. This freedom allows participants to reassess their decision

or discontinue their involvement if they experience unexpected side effects or personal concerns.

Accessing Clinical Trials:

Access to clinical trials is facilitated through various means:

11. Referrals from Healthcare Providers: Oncologists or healthcare providers who are aware of ongoing clinical trials can refer eligible patients to relevant research teams. This ensures that patients have access to potential trial opportunities that align with their condition and treatment goals.

12. Clinical Trial Databases: Online databases and registries, such as C linicalTrials.gov or other institutional databases, provide information on ongoing clinical trials. Individuals can search for trials based on their cancer type, location, or eligibility criteria, enabling them to explore potential participation opportunities.

13. Patient Advocacy Groups: Patient advocacy

## The future of chemotherapy

Chemotherapy has long been a cornerstone of cancer treatment, but ongoing advancements and research are shaping the future of this vital therapeutic approach. With emerging technologies, novel drug discoveries, and innovative treatment strategies, the landscape of chemotherapy is continuously evolving to improve patient outcomes and enhance the quality of life for individuals affected by cancer. This chapter explores the exciting possibilities and future directions of chemotherapy, providing factual information and insights into the transformative potential of these advancements.

Precision Medicine and Personalized Approaches:

Precision medicine is revolutionizing the field of chemotherapy by tailoring treatment to individual patients' unique characteristics:

2. Biomarker Testing: Biomarker testing identifies specific genetic or molecular alterations in tumors that can guide treatment decisions. This enables the selection of targeted chemotherapy agents that are more likely to be effective against the specific genetic profile of a patient's cancer.

3. Genomic Profiling: Genomic profiling analyzes a patient's DNA to identify genetic variations that may influence treatment response. By understanding the genetic landscape of tumors, clinicians can develop personalized treatment strategies that maximize efficacy and minimize side effects.

4. Liquid Biopsies: Liquid biopsies, such as circulating tumor DNA analysis, allow for non-invasive monitoring of tumor characteristics and treatment response. These tests provide real-time information on genetic changes, allowing for dynamic treatment adjustments.

Targeted Therapies and Immunotherapy:

Targeted therapies and immunotherapy are transforming the field of chemotherapy, offering more precise and effective treatment options:

5. Targeted Therapies: Targeted therapies selectively inhibit specific molecules or pathways involved in tumor growth, minimizing damage to healthy cells. They are designed to disrupt the molecular drivers of cancer cells, resulting in higher response rates and improved outcomes.

6. Immunotherapy: Immunotherapy harnesses the power of the immune system to recognize and destroy cancer cells. Immune checkpoint inhibitors, chimeric antigen receptor (CAR) T-cell therapy, and cancer vaccines are among the innovative immunotherapeutic approaches that enhance the body's ability to fight cancer.

Nanotechnology and Drug Delivery Systems:

Nanotechnology has the potential to revolutionize chemotherapy by improving drug delivery and enhancing treatment efficacy:

7. Nanoparticle-Based Delivery Systems: Nanoparticles can be engineered to encapsulate chemotherapy drugs and specifically target tumor cells, reducing off-target toxicity and enhancing drug uptake. These delivery systems improve drug solubility, stability, and pharmacokinetics, optimizing therapeutic outcomes.

8. Localized Drug Delivery: Implantable devices or localized drug delivery systems can deliver chemotherapy directly to the tumor site, minimizing systemic side effects and improving treatment efficacy. These approaches also enable the sustained release of drugs over time, reducing the need for frequent administrations.

Combination Therapies:

The future of chemotherapy lies in the development of synergistic combination therapies:

9. Chemotherapy Combinations: Combining multiple chemotherapy agents with different mechanisms of action can improve treatment outcomes by targeting cancer cells through different pathways, minimizing drug resistance, and increasing response rates.

10. Multimodal Approaches: Integrating chemotherapy with other treatment modalities, such as surgery, radiation therapy, targeted therapies, or immunotherapy, can maximize treatment effectiveness. Multimodal approaches take advantage of the complementary benefits of different treatment modalities, offering a more comprehensive and personalized treatment plan.

Artificial Intelligence and Big Data Analytics:

Artificial intelligence (AI) and big data analytics are poised to revolutionize chemotherapy research and clinical decision-making:

11. Predictive Modeling: AI algorithms can analyze vast amounts of patient data, including genetic profiles, treatment history, and clinical outcomes, to generate predictive models. These models can help guide treatment decisions by identifying the most effective chemotherapy regimens for individual patients.

12. Treatment Response Monitoring: AI algorithms can analyze medical images, such as radiographs or PET scans, to assess treatment

Chapter Fifteen

# Targeted Therapy and Immunotherapy

Chemotherapy has long been a critical component of cancer treatment, but recent advancements in targeted therapy and immunotherapy are transforming the landscape of chemotherapy. These innovative approaches offer more precise and effective treatment options by directly targeting cancer cells or enhancing the body's immune response. This chapter explores the fascinating world of targeted therapy and immunotherapy in relation to chemotherapy, providing factual information and insights into their groundbreaking potential to revolutionize cancer care.

2. Targeted Therapy: A Precise Attack on Cancer Cells

Targeted therapy is a revolutionary approach that focuses on specific molecular targets or pathways that are essential for cancer cell growth and survival. Unlike traditional chemotherapy that affects both healthy and cancerous cells, targeted therapy selectively targets cancer cells, minimizing harm to normal tissues. Here are some key aspects of targeted therapy:

3. Molecular Targets: Targeted therapy drugs are designed to interfere with specific molecules or proteins involved in tumor growth, such as growth factor receptors or signal transduction pathways. By disrupting these targets, targeted therapy impedes cancer cell proliferation and survival.

4. Personalized Approach: Targeted therapy can be personalized based on the unique genetic makeup of an individual's tumor. Biomarker testing,

such as genomic profiling, helps identify specific genetic alterations that guide treatment decisions. This allows for tailored therapies that have a higher likelihood of success.

5. Improved Efficacy: Targeted therapies often demonstrate higher response rates and improved outcomes compared to traditional chemotherapy. By selectively targeting cancer cells, they can more effectively halt tumor progression and extend survival.

6. Examples of Targeted Therapies: Numerous targeted therapy drugs have been developed for different types of cancer. For instance, HER2-targeted therapies (e.g., trastuzumab) are effective in HER2-positive breast cancer, while BRAF inhibitors (e.g., vemurafenib) are used for BRAF-mutant melanoma.

7. Immunotherapy: Unleashing the Power of the Immune System

Immunotherapy is a transformative approach that harnesses the body's immune system to recognize and attack cancer cells. It boosts the immune response, enabling it to identify and eliminate tumor cells. Key aspects of immunotherapy include:

8. Immune Checkpoint Inhibitors: Immune checkpoint inhibitors block the proteins on cancer cells or immune cells that prevent immune responses from being too strong. By inhibiting these proteins (e.g., PD-1, PD-L1, CTLA-4), checkpoint inhibitors allow the immune system to mount a robust attack against cancer cells.

9. CAR-T Cell Therapy: Chimeric antigen receptor (CAR) T-cell therapy is a personalized immunotherapy approach. T cells are genetically modified to express a receptor that recognizes specific tumor antigens. When infused back into the patient, these CAR-T cells can effectively target and kill cancer cells.

10. Cancer Vaccines: Cancer vaccines aim to stimulate the immune system to recognize and destroy cancer cells. They can be used as preventive vaccines to prevent cancer development or therapeutic vaccines to boost the immune response against existing tumors.

11. Combination Approaches: Immunotherapy can also be combined with other treatment modalities, such as chemotherapy or targeted therapy, to enhance treatment effectiveness. These combinations take advantage of the complementary benefits of different therapies and improve overall response rates.

Advantages and Challenges of Targeted Therapy and Immunotherapy:

Targeted therapy and immunotherapy offer several advantages over traditional chemotherapy, but they also present unique challenges:

12. Increased Precision: Targeted therapy and immunotherapy provide more precise treatment by specifically targeting cancer cells or boosting the immune response against cancer. This precision reduces harm to healthy tissues and minimizes side effects.

13. Improved Response Rates: Targeted therapy and immunotherapy have shown remarkable response rates in specific types of cancers. Some patients achieve long-lasting remission or even

## How targeted therapy works

Targeted therapy has revolutionized the field of chemotherapy by providing a more precise and effective approach to cancer treatment. Unlike traditional chemotherapy, which affects both healthy and cancerous cells, targeted therapy specifically targets the unique molecular features of cancer cells. This chapter explores the fascinating world of targeted therapy in relation to chemotherapy, providing factual information and insights into how this innovative approach works to combat cancer.

Understanding Molecular Targets:

Targeted therapy is designed to interfere with specific molecules or pathways that are crucial for cancer cell growth and survival. By targeting these specific molecular features, targeted therapies disrupt the cancer cells' ability to proliferate and evade normal cellular mechanisms. Here are some key aspects of molecular targets:

2. Genetic Alterations: Genetic alterations, such as mutations or gene amplifications, can drive cancer development and progression. Targeted therapies often aim to counteract these specific genetic abnormalities.

3. Growth Factors and Receptors: Growth factors and their corresponding receptors play a critical role in cell signaling and growth regulation. Targeted therapies can block these receptors or inhibit the growth factors themselves, disrupting the signals that promote cancer cell growth.

4. Signal Transduction Pathways: Signal transduction pathways are intricate networks of molecules that transmit signals from the cell surface to the nucleus, influencing cell growth, survival, and proliferation. Targeted therapies often aim to interrupt these pathways to halt cancer cell growth.

Modes of Action in Targeted Therapy:

Targeted therapy employs different modes of action to interfere with cancer cell growth and survival. Here are some common mechanisms of action:

5. Inhibition of Receptors: Targeted therapies can bind to specific receptors on cancer cells, preventing the binding of growth factors and the

subsequent activation of signaling pathways. This blockade disrupts the signals that promote cancer cell growth.

6. Small Molecule Inhibitors: Small molecule inhibitors are drugs that interfere with specific molecules involved in cancer cell growth. These drugs can be taken orally and are designed to inhibit the activity of specific enzymes or signaling molecules that are crucial for cancer cell survival.

7. Monoclonal Antibodies: Monoclonal antibodies are laboratory-produced molecules that specifically target cancer cells. They can bind to receptors on the cancer cell surface, marking them for destruction by the immune system or inhibiting their growth and survival.

8. Apoptosis Induction: Apoptosis is programmed cell death, a natural process that eliminates damaged or unwanted cells. Some targeted therapies can trigger apoptosis in cancer cells, leading to their destruction.

Biomarker Testing and Personalized Treatment:

Biomarker testing plays a crucial role in identifying patients who are most likely to benefit from targeted therapies. Biomarkers are specific characteristics or molecules that can be detected in a patient's tumor. Here are some important considerations:

9. Genetic Testing: Genetic testing analyzes the DNA of a patient's tumor to identify specific genetic alterations that can guide treatment decisions. For example, the presence of specific gene mutations may indicate eligibility for targeted therapy.

10. Companion Diagnostic Tests: Companion diagnostic tests are often developed alongside targeted therapies to identify patients who are most likely to benefit from a particular treatment. These tests detect specific biomarkers associated with the mechanism of action of the targeted therapy.

11. Personalized Treatment Decisions: Based on the results of biomarker testing, oncologists can make informed decisions about the most appropriate targeted therapy for an individual patient. This personalized approach maximizes treatment efficacy and reduces unnecessary side effects.

Advantages and Limitations of Targeted Therapy:

Targeted therapy offers several advantages over traditional chemotherapy, but it also has certain limitations:

12. Increased Precision: Targeted therapy specifically targets cancer cells, sparing healthy cells and minimizing side effects associated with traditional chemotherapy.

13. Higher Response Rates: Targeted therapy can achieve high response rates in patients with specific genetic

## The role of immunotherapy in cancer treatment

Immunotherapy has emerged as a groundbreaking approach in cancer treatment, revolutionizing the field of chemotherapy. Unlike traditional chemotherapy, which directly targets cancer cells, immunotherapy harnesses the body's immune system to recognize and eliminate cancer cells. This chapter explores the captivating role of immunotherapy in cancer treatment, providing factual information and insights into its transformative potential in conjunction with chemotherapy.

Understanding the Immune System's Role:

The immune system plays a crucial role in defending the body against pathogens, including cancer cells. However, cancer cells can develop mechanisms to evade detection and destruction by the immune system. Immunotherapy aims to enhance the immune response against cancer cells by various mechanisms. Here are some key aspects:

2. Immune Checkpoints: Immune checkpoint proteins, such as programmed cell death protein 1 (PD-1) and its ligand PD-L1, regulate the immune response. Cancer cells can exploit these checkpoints to evade immune detection. Immunotherapy targets these checkpoints, blocking the interaction between PD-1 and PD-L1, thereby reactivating the immune response against cancer cells.

3. Tumor-Infiltrating Lymphocytes: Tumor-infiltrating lymphocytes (TILs) are immune cells that infiltrate the tumor microenvironment. Immunotherapy aims to enhance the activity and effectiveness of TILs in recognizing and destroying cancer cells.

4. Recognition of Cancer-Specific Antigens: Cancer cells often express specific antigens that are not present in healthy cells. Immunotherapy stimulates the immune system to recognize these cancer-specific antigens, leading to targeted destruction of cancer cells while sparing normal cells.

Types of Immunotherapy:

Immunotherapy encompasses a range of approaches that harness the immune system to fight cancer. Here are some notable types of immunotherapy:

5. Immune Checkpoint Inhibitors: Immune checkpoint inhibitors (ICIs) are designed to block the inhibitory signals that cancer cells use to evade immune detection. By inhibiting proteins such as PD-1 or PD-L1, ICIs reinvigorate the immune response, allowing immune cells to recognize and destroy cancer cells more effectively.

6. CAR-T Cell Therapy: Chimeric antigen receptor (CAR) T-cell therapy involves engineering a patient's own T cells to express specific receptors

that recognize cancer cells. These modified T cells are then infused back into the patient's body, where they can effectively target and eliminate cancer cells.

7. Tumor Vaccines: Tumor vaccines stimulate the immune system to recognize and attack cancer cells. They can be composed of cancer-specific antigens, dendritic cells, or immune stimulatory molecules that promote an immune response against the tumor.

8. Adoptive Cell Transfer: Adoptive cell transfer involves isolating and expanding a patient's own T cells with tumor recognition capabilities. These T cells are then infused back into the patient, increasing the number of tumor-fighting immune cells.

Synergy with Chemotherapy:

Immunotherapy and chemotherapy can complement each other, leading to improved treatment outcomes. Here are some ways in which immunotherapy and chemotherapy can work synergistically:

9. Enhanced Response Rates: Combining immunotherapy with chemotherapy can increase the response rates in certain cancers. Chemotherapy can create an environment that exposes cancer cells to the immune system, making them more susceptible to immunotherapy.

10. Immunogenic Cell Death: Chemotherapy-induced cell death can release tumor antigens, activating the immune system to recognize and target cancer cells. This process, known as immunogenic cell death, can synergize with immunotherapy, further enhancing the immune response against cancer.

11. Modulating the Tumor Microenvironment: Chemotherapy can modify the tumor microenvironment, making it more favorable for the immune system to recognize and attack cancer cells. This

## Combination therapies

Combination therapies have emerged as a potent strategy in the field of chemotherapy, harnessing the power of multiple treatment modalities to combat cancer. By combining different therapeutic approaches, such as chemotherapy with targeted therapy, immunotherapy, or radiation therapy, researchers have unlocked new avenues for improved treatment outcomes. This chapter explores the intriguing world of combination therapies in relation to chemotherapy, providing factual information and insights into the exciting potential of synergistic treatment approaches.

2. Synergy: Enhancing Treatment Efficacy

Synergy refers to the enhanced effectiveness achieved when two or more treatment modalities are combined. In the context of chemotherapy, combination therapies aim to maximize treatment outcomes through various mechanisms:

3. Improved Tumor Response: Different treatment modalities can target cancer cells through complementary pathways, leading to a more comprehensive attack on the tumor. This enhanced attack can result in improved tumor response rates, shrinkage, and control.

4. Overcoming Drug Resistance: Cancer cells can develop resistance to chemotherapy drugs over time. Combination therapies offer the opportunity to counteract drug resistance by targeting multiple vulnerabilities of the cancer cells simultaneously. This approach reduces the likelihood of cancer cells evading treatment and improves overall response rates.

5. Synergistic Effects: Certain treatment combinations exhibit synergistic effects, where the combined action of the therapies is more potent than

the sum of their individual effects. This synergy can lead to enhanced cell death, inhibition of tumor growth, and improved treatment outcomes.

Types of Combination Therapies

Combination therapies in chemotherapy encompass a range of approaches, each with its own unique benefits and mechanisms of action. Some notable types include:

6. Chemotherapy with Targeted Therapy: Combining chemotherapy with targeted therapy, which specifically targets molecules or pathways involved in cancer cell growth, can enhance treatment efficacy. Targeted therapies can complement chemotherapy by inhibiting specific signaling pathways, reducing drug resistance, and improving response rates.

7. Chemotherapy with Immunotherapy: The combination of chemotherapy with immunotherapy aims to enhance the immune system's ability to recognize and attack cancer cells. Chemotherapy can create a more favorable environment by stimulating the release of tumor antigens and modulating the tumor microenvironment. Immunotherapy then works in synergy by activating and boosting the immune response against cancer cells.

8. Chemotherapy with Radiation Therapy: Combining chemotherapy with radiation therapy, known as chemoradiation, can be highly effective in certain cancers. Chemotherapy can sensitize cancer cells to radiation, making them more susceptible to its damaging effects. This approach enhances the local control of tumors and can be curative in some cases.

Advantages of Combination Therapies

Combination therapies offer several advantages over single-modality treatments in chemotherapy:

9. Increased Treatment Efficacy: By targeting cancer cells through multiple mechanisms, combination therapies can improve treatment response rates, reduce tumor size, and increase overall survival. This enhanced efficacy is particularly valuable in aggressive or advanced-stage cancers.

10. Reduced Drug Resistance: Cancer cells can develop resistance to single chemotherapy drugs over time. Combining different drugs with distinct mechanisms of action reduces the likelihood of resistance development, as cancer cells would need to simultaneously overcome the vulnerabilities targeted by multiple agents.

11. Minimized Toxicity: Combination therapies can sometimes allow for reduced individual drug dosages, minimizing the toxicity and side effects associated with higher doses of a single drug. By synergizing the effects of different treatments, lower doses may achieve the same therapeutic outcome with fewer adverse effects.

Challenges and Considerations

While combination therapies hold great promise, several challenges and considerations exist:

12. Increased Toxicity: Combining different therapies can potentially increase the overall toxicity experienced by the patient. The cumulative side effects of multiple treatments must be carefully managed to ensure optimal patient tolerability and well-being.

Treatment Sequencing and Timing:

Chapter Sixteen

# Chemotherapy and Palliative Care

Chemotherapy, a cornerstone of cancer treatment, aims to eradicate or control cancer cells. However, it is important to recognize that the goals of cancer treatment extend beyond survival alone. Palliative care plays a crucial role in supporting patients throughout their cancer journey, focusing on enhancing quality of life and managing symptoms. This chapter explores the intersection of chemotherapy and palliative care, shedding light on the valuable role of palliative care in improving the well-being of patients undergoing chemotherapy.

2. Palliative Care: A Holistic Approach

Palliative care is a multidisciplinary approach that aims to optimize the quality of life for individuals facing serious illnesses, including cancer. It addresses physical, emotional, social, and spiritual needs, providing support to patients and their families. Here are some key aspects of palliative care:

3. Symptom Management: Palliative care focuses on alleviating symptoms associated with cancer and its treatment. This includes the management of pain, nausea, fatigue, and other side effects of chemotherapy. By effectively controlling symptoms, palliative care enhances patients' comfort and overall well-being.

4. Emotional Support: Cancer diagnosis and treatment can evoke a wide range of emotions, including anxiety, fear, and sadness. Palliative care pro-

fessionals offer emotional support, providing a safe space for patients to express their feelings and cope with the emotional challenges they may face.

5. Communication and Shared Decision-Making: Palliative care teams facilitate open and honest communication between patients, families, and healthcare providers. They ensure that patients understand their treatment options, potential benefits, and risks, empowering them to actively participate in shared decision-making regarding their care.

6. Continuity of Care: Palliative care teams collaborate closely with oncologists and other healthcare providers to ensure seamless coordination of care. They provide support throughout the cancer journey, from diagnosis through treatment, survivorship, or end-of-life care.

Integrating Palliative Care with Chemotherapy

Chemotherapy and palliative care can and should work together to provide comprehensive support to patients. Integrating palliative care with chemotherapy offers several benefits:

7. Enhanced Symptom Management: Chemotherapy often causes side effects that can significantly impact a patient's quality of life. Palliative care specialists have expertise in managing these symptoms, offering strategies to mitigate chemotherapy-related side effects such as nausea, pain, and fatigue.

8. Emotional and Psychosocial Support: The emotional toll of chemotherapy can be immense, affecting patients and their families. Palliative care teams provide counseling, support groups, and other psychosocial interventions to help individuals cope with the emotional challenges associated with cancer treatment.

9. Improved Communication and Decision-Making: Palliative care professionals facilitate open and honest communication among patients, fam-

ilies, and healthcare providers. They help patients understand their treatment options, potential outcomes, and assist in making informed decisions aligned with their goals and values.

10. Advanced Care Planning: Palliative care teams assist patients in discussing and documenting their preferences for future medical care, including end-of-life decisions. By engaging in advance care planning, patients have the opportunity to express their wishes, ensuring their treatment aligns with their values and goals.

Palliative Care Across the Cancer Continuum

Palliative care is not limited to end-of-life care. It can be integrated at any stage of the cancer continuum, including during active chemotherapy treatment. Here are some key considerations:

11. Early Integration: Research suggests that early integration of palliative care alongside chemotherapy can positively impact patient outcomes. Early involvement allows for proactive symptom management and improves patients' overall quality of life.

12. Survivorship Care: Palliative care continues to play a role in survivorship care, addressing the physical and emotional needs of cancer survivors. By providing ongoing support and monitoring for potential late effects or recurrence, palliative care teams ensure holistic care even

## The role of palliative care in cancer treatment

Cancer treatment goes beyond eradicating or controlling cancer cells. It encompasses the holistic care of patients, focusing on their physical, emotional, and psychosocial well-being. Palliative care plays a vital role in cancer treatment, working alongside chemotherapy to provide comprehensive support and improve the quality of life for patients. This chapter explores the valuable role of palliative care in cancer treatment, with a specific focus on its relationship with chemotherapy.

Understanding Palliative Care:

Palliative care is a specialized form of medical care that focuses on improving the quality of life for patients facing serious illnesses, such as cancer. It addresses the physical, emotional, social, and spiritual needs of patients and their families throughout the cancer journey. Key aspects of palliative care include:

2. Symptom Management: Palliative care aims to alleviate symptoms associated with cancer and its treatment. This includes managing pain, nausea, fatigue, and other side effects of chemotherapy. By providing effective symptom management, palliative care enhances patients' comfort and well-being.

3. Communication and Shared Decision-Making: Palliative care teams facilitate open and honest communication between patients, families, and healthcare providers. They help patients understand their treatment options, potential benefits, and risks, empowering them to actively participate in shared decision-making regarding their care.

4. Emotional and Psychosocial Support: Cancer diagnosis and treatment can evoke a wide range of emotions, including anxiety, fear, and sadness. Palliative care professionals provide emotional support, counseling, and psychosocial interventions to help patients and families cope with the emotional challenges of cancer.

5. Advance Care Planning: Palliative care teams engage in advance care planning discussions, assisting patients in expressing their healthcare preferences and goals. This ensures that treatment aligns with their values and wishes, including decisions regarding end-of-life care.

Integration of Palliative Care and Chemotherapy:

Palliative care and chemotherapy are not mutually exclusive; rather, they work hand in hand to provide comprehensive support to patients. Integration of palliative care with chemotherapy offers several benefits:

6. Improved Symptom Management: Chemotherapy often causes side effects that can significantly impact a patient's quality of life. Palliative care specialists have expertise in managing these symptoms, offering strategies to mitigate chemotherapy-related side effects such as nausea, pain, and fatigue.

7. Emotional and Psychosocial Support: The emotional toll of cancer and chemotherapy can be immense, affecting patients and their families. Palliative care teams provide counseling, support groups, and other interventions to help individuals cope with the emotional challenges associated with cancer treatment.

8. Communication and Decision-Making: Palliative care professionals facilitate open and honest communication among patients, families, and healthcare providers. They help patients understand their treatment options, potential outcomes, and assist in making informed decisions aligned with their goals and values.

9. Continuity of Care: Palliative care teams collaborate closely with oncologists and other healthcare providers to ensure seamless coordination of care. They provide support throughout the cancer journey, from diagnosis through treatment, survivorship, or end-of-life care.

Palliative Care Throughout the Cancer Continuum:

Palliative care is not limited to end-of-life care. It is beneficial at any stage of the cancer continuum, including during active chemotherapy treatment. Here are some key considerations:

10. Early Integration: Research suggests that early integration of palliative care alongside chemotherapy can positively impact patient outcomes. Early involvement allows for proactive symptom management, improves patients' overall quality of life, and helps them better navigate their cancer journey.

11. Survivorship Care: Palliative care continues to play a role in survivorship care, addressing the physical and emotional needs of cancer survivors. By providing ongoing support, monitoring for potential late effects or recurrence, and promoting healthy survivorship, palliative care teams

## Managing pain and other symptoms

1. Managing Pain and Other Symptoms: Enhancing Comfort during Chemotherapy

Chemotherapy, a key component of cancer treatment, can bring about various side effects that impact a patient's quality of life. Pain and other symptoms associated with chemotherapy can be challenging to manage, but advancements in supportive care have significantly improved the management of these issues. This chapter explores the importance of effectively managing pain and other symptoms in relation to chemotherapy, providing factual information and insights into strategies and interventions that enhance patients' comfort during treatment.

Understanding Chemotherapy Side Effects:

Chemotherapy drugs work by targeting rapidly dividing cells, including cancer cells. However, they can also affect healthy cells, leading to a range of side effects. Here are some common symptoms experienced during chemotherapy:

2. Pain: Chemotherapy can cause pain in various forms, such as headaches, muscle pain, joint pain, and nerve pain (neuropathy). Pain can significantly impact a patient's daily activities and overall well-being.

3. Nausea and Vomiting: Chemotherapy-induced nausea and vomiting (CINV) are common side effects that can cause significant discomfort and affect a patient's ability to eat, leading to malnutrition and dehydration.

4. Fatigue: Cancer-related fatigue is a persistent and overwhelming feeling of tiredness that can interfere with a patient's ability to carry out daily activities and impact their overall quality of life.

5. Gastrointestinal Symptoms: Chemotherapy can cause digestive issues, including diarrhea, constipation, and changes in appetite. These symptoms can lead to nutritional deficiencies and negatively affect a patient's well-being.

Multidimensional Approach to Symptom Management:

Effectively managing pain and other symptoms during chemotherapy requires a multidimensional approach that addresses the physical, emotional, and psychosocial aspects of patient care. Here are some key strategies and interventions:

6. Medications: Pharmacological interventions play a crucial role in symptom management during chemotherapy. Analgesics, such as opioids and nonsteroidal anti-inflammatory drugs (NSAIDs), can help alleviate pain. Antiemetic medications are prescribed to control chemotherapy-induced nausea and vomiting. Other medications, such as laxatives or antidiarrheals, can address gastrointestinal symptoms.

7. Integrative Therapies: Complementary and integrative therapies, such as acupuncture, massage therapy, yoga, and relaxation techniques, can provide relief from pain, nausea, and fatigue. These therapies can be used

in conjunction with conventional treatments to enhance symptom management and improve overall well-being.

8. Nutritional Support: Proper nutrition is crucial during chemotherapy to support the body's healing process and mitigate treatment-related side effects. Dietary modifications, such as consuming small, frequent meals and avoiding trigger foods, can help manage gastrointestinal symptoms. In some cases, nutritional supplements may be recommended to maintain adequate nutrient intake.

9. Psychological and Emotional Support: Psychological support is essential for patients undergoing chemotherapy. Counseling, support groups, and cognitive-behavioral therapy can help patients cope with pain, anxiety, and depression. Mind-body techniques, such as meditation and mindfulness, can also promote emotional well-being.

10. Exercise and Physical Activity: Regular exercise and physical activity, tailored to individual capabilities, can improve overall well-being, reduce fatigue, and alleviate pain. Consultation with healthcare providers is crucial to determine the appropriate level of exercise and ensure safety during chemotherapy.

Individualized Symptom Management:

Every patient's experience with chemotherapy and associated symptoms is unique. Individualized symptom management ensures that interventions are tailored to the specific needs and preferences of each patient. Here are some important considerations:

11. Assessment and Communication: Regular assessment of symptoms and open communication between patients and healthcare providers are essential for effective symptom management. Patients should commu-

nicate any changes or new symptoms experienced, allowing healthcare providers to address them promptly.

12. Treatment Modification: Depending on the severity of symptoms, modifications to the chemotherapy regimen may be considered

## End-of-life care and support

End-of-life care is a vital component of cancer treatment, ensuring that patients receive compassionate support and optimal comfort during their final stages of life. While chemotherapy aims to treat and control cancer, it is crucial to recognize when the focus should shift towards providing palliative and supportive care to maintain dignity and quality of life. This chapter explores the importance of end-of-life care and support in the context of chemotherapy, providing factual information and insights into the interventions and resources available to enhance the well-being of patients and their loved ones during this challenging period.

Recognizing the Transition to End-of-Life Care:

End-of-life care becomes relevant when the goals of treatment shift from curative or disease control to the management of symptoms and the provision of emotional and spiritual support. In the context of chemotherapy, several factors indicate the need to consider end-of-life care:

2. Disease Progression: When cancer reaches an advanced stage and chemotherapy is no longer effective in controlling the disease, the focus may shift towards maximizing comfort and quality of life.

3. Treatment Preferences: Patients may express a desire to discontinue chemotherapy or forgo further aggressive treatment in favor of palliative care aimed at symptom management and support.

4. Prognosis: The healthcare team's evaluation of the patient's prognosis, based on factors such as the progression of the disease and the response to treatment, can guide the transition to end-of-life care.

Goals of End-of-Life Care:

End-of-life care focuses on providing physical, emotional, and spiritual support to patients and their families during the final stages of life. Here are the key goals of end-of-life care:

5. Symptom Management: Effective pain and symptom management is paramount in ensuring the patient's comfort. Medications, such as opioids and other analgesics, are prescribed to alleviate pain. Other interventions, such as antiemetics for nausea and vomiting, help manage distressing symptoms associated with chemotherapy and cancer.

6. Emotional Support: End-of-life care addresses the emotional needs of patients and their loved ones. Social workers, counselors, and psychologists provide counseling and support to navigate the complex emotions and challenges associated with the end of life.

7. Communication and Shared Decision-Making: Open and compassionate communication between patients, families, and healthcare providers is essential. Discussions about treatment options, goals of care, and advance care planning enable patients to make informed decisions and express their wishes regarding their end-of-life care.

8. Holistic Care: End-of-life care recognizes the importance of attending to the spiritual and psychosocial needs of patients. Chaplains, spiritual care providers, and palliative care teams offer guidance, counseling, and support to patients and families based on their individual beliefs and preferences.

Hospice Care:

Hospice care is a specialized form of end-of-life care that provides comprehensive support and comfort to patients with a life-limiting illness. Hospice care can be beneficial during and after chemotherapy, focusing on enhancing the quality of life during the final stages of the disease. Key aspects of hospice care include:

9. Comfort-Centered Approach: Hospice care emphasizes pain and symptom management, ensuring that patients are as comfortable as possible. A multidisciplinary team collaborates to address physical, emotional, and spiritual needs.

10. Home-Based Care: Hospice care can be provided at home, allowing patients to remain in a familiar and supportive environment surrounded by their loved ones. This approach offers a sense of continuity and promotes a dignified and peaceful end-of-life experience.

11. Psychosocial Support: Hospice care provides emotional and psychosocial support to patients and their families. Counseling, bereavement support, and respite care for caregivers are integral components of hospice services.

12. Care Coordination: Hospice care

Chapter Seventeen

# Survivorship and Life After Chemotherapy

Survivorship marks an important milestone in the cancer journey, signifying the completion of chemotherapy and the transition into life after treatment. For many individuals, this phase can bring about a mix of emotions and challenges as they adjust to a "new normal." This chapter explores the concept of survivorship and life after chemotherapy, providing factual information and insights into the various aspects of survivorship care, empowering individuals to navigate this phase with resilience and embrace a fulfilling life beyond cancer.

Understanding Survivorship:

Survivorship encompasses the period after the completion of cancer treatment, including chemotherapy. It recognizes that the impact of cancer extends beyond the physical aspects of the disease and treatment, encompassing emotional, psychological, and social aspects as well. Key aspects of survivorship include:

2. Emotional Adjustment: The transition from active treatment to survivorship can be emotionally challenging. Individuals may experience a range of emotions, including relief, fear of recurrence, anxiety, and uncertainty about the future. Acknowledging and addressing these emotions is essential for well-being.

3. Physical Recovery: While chemotherapy can cause short-term and long-term side effects, survivorship is characterized by physical healing

and recovery. Managing treatment-related symptoms, such as fatigue, neuropathy, and changes in body composition, becomes a key focus during this phase.

4. Follow-Up Care: Regular follow-up visits and screenings are essential to monitor for potential cancer recurrence or the development of late effects related to treatment. These appointments provide an opportunity to address any concerns, manage long-term side effects, and promote overall health and well-being.

Embracing Life After Chemotherapy:

Life after chemotherapy presents unique opportunities and challenges. Embracing this phase involves several key considerations:

5. Emotional Well-being: Emotional support remains crucial during survivorship. Engaging in self-care practices, seeking counseling or support groups, and connecting with other cancer survivors can help individuals navigate the emotional challenges and foster a sense of resilience.

6. Physical Rehabilitation: Physical recovery may involve rehabilitation to address any lingering treatment-related side effects. Exercise, physical therapy, and rehabilitation programs can help restore strength, manage fatigue, and enhance overall physical well-being.

7. Healthy Lifestyle Choices: Adopting a healthy lifestyle becomes paramount during survivorship. Engaging in regular physical activity, following a balanced diet, avoiding tobacco and excessive alcohol consumption, and maintaining a healthy weight contribute to long-term health and well-being.

8. Long-Term Effects Management: Some individuals may experience long-term effects of chemotherapy or late effects related to cancer treat-

ment. Regular communication with healthcare providers and active management of these effects are crucial to minimizing their impact on daily life.

Survivorship Care Planning:

Survivorship care planning involves the development of a comprehensive care plan tailored to each individual's unique needs. Key components of survivorship care planning include:

9. Survivorship Care Plan: A survivorship care plan is a written document that summarizes the individual's cancer diagnosis, treatment received, potential long-term effects, and recommendations for follow-up care. It serves as a roadmap for ongoing care and communication between the individual and their healthcare team.

10. Follow-Up Care: Regular follow-up visits are an essential aspect of survivorship care. These visits allow healthcare providers to monitor for any signs of recurrence, manage treatment-related side effects, and address any concerns or questions the individual may have.

11. Health Promotion: Survivorship care emphasizes health promotion and disease prevention. This includes educating individuals about healthy lifestyle choices, encouraging cancer screenings as appropriate, and providing resources for managing long-term effects.

12. Transitioning Support: During the transition from active treatment to survivorship, individuals may require additional support. Survivorship programs, support groups, and counseling services can play a pivotal role in addressing the unique challenges and fostering a sense of community and

## Long-term effects of chemotherapy

Chemotherapy is a powerful treatment modality that has significantly improved cancer outcomes for many patients. While chemotherapy can be life-saving, it can also have long-term effects on both physical and psychological well-being. This chapter explores the long-term effects of chemotherapy, shedding light on the potential challenges individuals may face during their journey to survivorship. By providing factual information and insights, this piece aims to empower individuals to proactively manage these effects and embrace a fulfilling life beyond cancer.

Understanding Long-term Effects:

Long-term effects refer to the physical and psychological changes that persist or arise after the completion of chemotherapy treatment. These effects can vary depending on the type of chemotherapy drugs used, the dosage, and individual factors. It is important to note that not all individuals will experience long-term effects, and the severity and duration can vary widely. Common long-term effects include:

2. Physical Effects: Chemotherapy can cause physical changes, such as fatigue, peripheral neuropathy (nerve damage leading to numbness or tingling), cognitive dysfunction (chemo brain), changes in fertility, cardiotoxicity, and secondary cancers.

3. Emotional and Psychological Effects: Cancer and its treatment can have a significant impact on mental health. Many individuals experience anxiety, depression, fear of recurrence, post-traumatic stress disorder (PTSD), and body image issues.

Managing Physical Long-term Effects:

Managing physical long-term effects requires a comprehensive approach that addresses each individual's unique needs. Here are some strategies and interventions to consider:

4. Fatigue Management: Fatigue is a common long-term effect. Maintaining a balanced lifestyle, engaging in regular physical activity, managing stress, and conserving energy through prioritization and delegation of tasks can help manage fatigue.

5. Peripheral Neuropathy: Peripheral neuropathy can affect the hands and feet, leading to numbness, tingling, or pain. Medications, physical therapy, occupational therapy, and alternative therapies such as acupuncture may help alleviate symptoms.

6. Cognitive Dysfunction: Cognitive changes, often referred to as chemo brain, can affect memory, concentration, and executive functions. Strategies such as using memory aids, maintaining a structured routine, engaging in cognitive exercises, and seeking cognitive rehabilitation can help manage these challenges.

7. Cardiotoxicity Management: Regular cardiovascular monitoring and adopting a heart-healthy lifestyle, including a balanced diet, regular exercise, smoking cessation, and stress management, are essential in mitigating the risk of cardiotoxicity.

8. Fertility Preservation and Family Planning: Chemotherapy can impact fertility, leading to temporary or permanent infertility. Discussing fertility preservation options before starting treatment and exploring alternatives such as adoption or assisted reproductive technologies can help individuals plan for their future family-building goals.

9. Secondary Cancer Screening: Certain chemotherapy drugs increase the risk of developing secondary cancers. Regular screenings and close monitoring for signs and symptoms of secondary cancers are important for early detection and prompt treatment.

Addressing Emotional and Psychological Long-term Effects:

The emotional and psychological impact of chemotherapy can persist long after treatment completion. Here are some strategies to address these effects:

10. Psychological Support: Seeking support from mental health professionals, joining support groups, and participating in counseling or therapy sessions can provide valuable emotional support and tools for coping with anxiety, depression, PTSD, and fear of recurrence.

11. Lifestyle Changes: Engaging in self-care practices such as regular exercise, healthy eating, mindfulness meditation, and stress reduction techniques can support mental well-being and overall quality of life.

12. Body Image and Self-esteem: Changes in physical appearance due to chemotherapy can affect body image and self-esteem. Exploring support groups, counseling, or body-positive initiatives can help individuals navigate these challenges and promote self-acceptance and self-compassion.

Survivorship Care:

Survivorship care is essential in

## Follow-up care and monitoring

Chemotherapy is a cornerstone of cancer treatment, helping patients combat the disease and achieve remission. However, the journey to recovery does not end with the completion of chemotherapy. Follow-up care and monitoring play a crucial role in ensuring long-term wellness, detecting potential recurrence or late effects, and supporting survivors on their path to health. This chapter explores the significance of follow-up care and monitoring in relation to chemotherapy, highlighting key aspects and providing valuable insights to empower individuals in sustaining their well-being beyond treatment.

The Importance of Follow-Up Care:

Follow-up care involves regular medical check-ups and assessments after completing chemotherapy treatment. It serves multiple purposes, including:

2. Early Detection of Recurrence: Follow-up appointments enable healthcare providers to monitor for any signs of cancer recurrence or relapse. Early detection significantly improves the chances of successful intervention and treatment.

3. Management of Late Effects: Some individuals may experience long-term effects related to chemotherapy or late effects associated with cancer treatment. Follow-up care provides an opportunity to address and manage these effects, ensuring optimal quality of life for survivors.

4. Addressing Physical and Emotional Concerns: Follow-up visits allow survivors to discuss any physical or emotional concerns they may have. This may include ongoing symptoms, potential side effects, or psychosocial challenges. Healthcare providers can offer guidance, support, and referrals as needed.

Elements of Follow-Up Care:

Follow-up care is tailored to each individual's specific needs, treatment history, and cancer type. Here are some key elements commonly included in follow-up care:

5. Medical History Review: Healthcare providers will review the patient's medical history, including details of the cancer diagnosis, treatment received (such as specific chemotherapy agents), and any other relevant medical information.

6. Physical Examination: A comprehensive physical examination is conducted to assess the patient's overall health, monitor vital signs, and identify any physical changes or potential signs of recurrence.

7. Diagnostic Tests: Depending on the individual's cancer type and treatment history, various diagnostic tests may be ordered, such as blood tests, imaging studies (e.g., CT scans, X-rays), or specific tumor markers to evaluate response to treatment and detect any signs of recurrence.

8. Survivorship Care Plan: A survivorship care plan is developed in collaboration with the patient and their healthcare team. This document outlines the individual's treatment history, potential long-term effects, recommended follow-up schedule, and strategies for promoting overall health and well-being.

9. Health Promotion and Education: Follow-up care includes health promotion and education. Patients are provided with information about healthy lifestyle choices, preventive measures, and resources to support their physical and emotional well-being.

Frequency and Duration of Follow-Up:

The frequency and duration of follow-up appointments vary depending on factors such as cancer type, stage, treatment received, and individual risk factors. In general, the following considerations apply:

10. Initial Period: In the first few years following chemotherapy completion, follow-up visits are often more frequent, typically every few months. This allows healthcare providers to closely monitor the patient's recovery, assess treatment response, and address any immediate concerns.

11. Transition to Long-Term Follow-Up: As time passes without evidence of recurrence or significant late effects, the frequency of follow-up visits

may decrease. However, regular check-ups are still recommended, usually transitioning to annual visits over time.

12. Lifelong Monitoring: For some cancer survivors, lifelong monitoring may be necessary due to a higher risk of recurrence or late effects. This is especially true for certain cancer types, such as breast, colon, or hematological cancers. In such cases, healthcare providers will develop an individualized follow-up plan to ensure ongoing surveillance and support.

Survivor's Active Role in Follow-Up Care:

Active involvement in follow-up care empowers survivors to take ownership of their

## Embracing life after treatment

Completing chemotherapy treatment is a significant milestone in the cancer journey. It marks the end of a challenging chapter and opens the door to a new phase of life filled with hope, possibilities, and the opportunity to embrace a vibrant and fulfilling future. This chapter explores the importance of embracing life after treatment, providing factual information, insights, and practical tips to empower individuals to navigate this transformative period with resilience, optimism, and a renewed sense of purpose.

The Transition to Life After Treatment:

Transitioning from active treatment to life after chemotherapy can bring about a mix of emotions and challenges. Here are some key aspects to consider:

2. Emotional Healing: It is essential to acknowledge and address the emotional impact of the cancer experience. Allow yourself to grieve, reflect,

and process your emotions. Seek support from loved ones, counseling, or support groups to help navigate the complexities of this transition.

3. Physical Recovery: While chemotherapy can cause short-term and long-term side effects, life after treatment is characterized by physical healing and recovery. Be patient with yourself as you regain strength and stamina. Engage in regular exercise, follow a nutritious diet, and prioritize self-care to support your overall well-being.

4. Fear of Recurrence: Fear of cancer recurrence is common among cancer survivors. Acknowledge these concerns but do not let them overshadow your ability to embrace life. Focus on adopting a positive mindset, engaging in healthy habits, and taking proactive steps to manage your health.

Nurturing Physical and Mental Well-being:

Life after treatment provides an opportunity to prioritize your physical and mental well-being. Here are some strategies to embrace:

5. Healthy Lifestyle Choices: Adopt a balanced and nutritious diet, rich in fruits, vegetables, whole grains, and lean proteins. Limit processed foods, sugary drinks, and alcohol consumption. Stay hydrated, avoid smoking, and practice sun protection. These lifestyle choices can support your overall health and reduce the risk of recurrence.

6. Regular Exercise: Engage in regular physical activity that suits your abilities and preferences. Consult with your healthcare team to determine appropriate exercises. Whether it's walking, swimming, yoga, or strength training, regular exercise can enhance your physical strength, boost your mood, and improve your overall quality of life.

7. Restorative Sleep: Prioritize restful sleep and establish a consistent sleep routine. Create a relaxing environment, limit exposure to screens

before bed, and practice relaxation techniques such as deep breathing or meditation to promote quality sleep.

8. Mental and Emotional Well-being: Focus on nurturing your mental health by practicing self-care activities that bring you joy and relaxation. Engage in hobbies, spend time with loved ones, seek support from professional counselors or therapists, and practice mindfulness or meditation to reduce stress and enhance emotional well-being.

Establishing a Supportive Network:

Building a strong support network is crucial in navigating life after treatment. Consider the following:

9. Communicate with Loved Ones: Share your feelings, concerns, and triumphs with trusted family members and friends. Allow them to support you emotionally and practically as you transition into this new phase.

10. Support Groups: Joining cancer survivor support groups or connecting with fellow survivors can provide a sense of community, understanding, and shared experiences. These groups offer valuable support, guidance, and the opportunity to learn from others who have walked a similar path.

11. Professional Support: Consider seeking the assistance of healthcare professionals, such as social workers, psychologists, or counselors, who specialize in survivorship care. They can provide guidance on managing emotional challenges, facilitate conversations about relationships, work, and lifestyle adjustments, and help you develop coping strategies for the journey ahead.

Setting Goals and Cultivating Purpose:

Embracing life after treatment involves rediscovering your passions, setting meaningful goals, and cultivating a sense of purpose.

Chapter Eighteen

# Caregivers and Support Systems

Chemotherapy treatment not only impacts the individuals undergoing it but also extends its effects to their caregivers and support systems. Caregivers play a vital role in providing physical, emotional, and practical support to their loved ones throughout the chemotherapy journey. This chapter explores the importance of caregivers and support systems in relation to chemotherapy, shedding light on their challenges, needs, and the available resources to empower them in their caregiving role.

The Role of Caregivers:

Caregivers are the unsung heroes of the chemotherapy journey, providing invaluable support to their loved ones facing cancer. Their role encompasses a range of responsibilities:

2. Practical Assistance: Caregivers often help with activities of daily living, such as transportation, meal preparation, medication management, and attending medical appointments. They provide essential physical support to ensure the well-being and comfort of the individual undergoing treatment.

3. Emotional Support: Caregivers offer a compassionate presence, listening ear, and empathetic understanding. They provide emotional support, offering reassurance, encouragement, and a source of strength during challenging times.

4. Advocacy: Caregivers advocate for their loved ones' needs, ensuring effective communication with healthcare providers, navigating the healthcare system, and helping to make informed decisions about treatment options.

5. Coordinating Care: Caregivers play a pivotal role in coordinating medical appointments, managing medications, organizing caregiving schedules, and maintaining open lines of communication between the individual and the healthcare team.

Challenges Faced by Caregivers:

Caregiving can be both rewarding and demanding, often presenting challenges that impact the caregiver's physical, emotional, and social well-being. Some common challenges faced by caregivers during chemotherapy include:

6. Emotional Strain: Witnessing a loved one go through the physical and emotional challenges of chemotherapy can be emotionally taxing. Caregivers may experience feelings of helplessness, stress, anxiety, and sadness. It is essential for caregivers to prioritize their own emotional well-being and seek support when needed.

7. Physical Demands: Caregiving responsibilities can be physically demanding, leading to fatigue and exhaustion. Long hours, sleep disturbances, and the need to balance caregiving with other responsibilities can take a toll on the caregiver's own health. It is crucial for caregivers to prioritize self-care and seek assistance when necessary.

8. Financial Burden: Chemotherapy treatment and related expenses can impose a financial burden on both the individual and the caregiver. Costs may include medical bills, transportation, accommodation, and additional

support services. Caregivers should explore available financial resources, insurance coverage, and support programs to alleviate the financial strain.

Building a Support System:

Recognizing the importance of building a strong support system is essential for both the individual undergoing chemotherapy and their caregivers. Here are some strategies for establishing and nurturing a support system:

9. Open Communication: Establish open and honest communication within the family and with healthcare professionals. Encourage dialogue, share concerns, and discuss expectations, ensuring everyone is on the same page regarding caregiving roles and responsibilities.

10. Family and Friends: Engage family members and close friends in the caregiving journey. Seek their assistance and support, whether it be through helping with tasks, offering emotional support, or providing respite care to allow the caregiver some time for self-care.

11. Support Groups: Caregiver support groups provide a safe space to connect with others who are going through similar experiences. These groups offer a sense of understanding, practical advice, and emotional support. Online support communities can also be a valuable resource, providing convenience and accessibility.

12. Professional Support: Seek guidance from healthcare professionals, social workers, or counselors who specialize in caregiver support. These professionals can offer coping strategies, education, and emotional support tailored to the caregiver's specific needs.

Respite

## The role of caregivers during treatment

Chemotherapy treatment can be physically and emotionally challenging for individuals battling cancer. During this time, caregivers play a vital role in providing the much-needed support and assistance. They serve as pillars of strength, offering physical, emotional, and practical help to their loved ones throughout the chemotherapy journey. This chapter explores the significant role of caregivers during treatment, highlighting their responsibilities, challenges, and the importance of self-care to ensure they can fulfill their caregiving role effectively.

Providing Physical Assistance:

Caregivers play a crucial role in providing physical assistance to individuals undergoing chemotherapy. Their responsibilities encompass a range of tasks:

2. Transportation: Caregivers ensure their loved ones get to and from medical appointments, chemotherapy sessions, and other necessary healthcare visits. They may also assist with running errands, picking up prescriptions, and managing transportation logistics.

3. Medication Management: Caregivers help with medication administration, ensuring that the prescribed chemotherapy drugs are taken correctly and on schedule. They may also handle the organization and tracking of medications, including managing any potential side effects.

4. Activities of Daily Living: Caregivers assist with activities of daily living, such as bathing, dressing, grooming, and meal preparation. They provide the necessary physical support to help their loved ones maintain their well-being and comfort during treatment.

Offering Emotional Support:

Emotional support is an essential aspect of a caregiver's role. During chemotherapy treatment, individuals may experience a range of emotions, including fear, anxiety, sadness, and uncertainty. Caregivers provide a supportive presence and offer emotional reassurance:

5. Active Listening: Caregivers lend a compassionate ear, allowing individuals to express their fears, concerns, and frustrations. They actively listen without judgment, providing a safe space for their loved ones to share their emotions and thoughts.

6. Providing Encouragement: Caregivers offer words of encouragement, reminding individuals of their strength and resilience. They provide emotional support and reinforce a positive mindset throughout the treatment process.

7. Coping Strategies: Caregivers help their loved ones develop and implement coping strategies to manage the emotional challenges of chemotherapy. These may include relaxation techniques, mindfulness exercises, or engaging in activities that bring joy and distraction.

Navigating the Healthcare System:

Caregivers play a crucial role in navigating the complex healthcare system, acting as advocates for their loved ones:

8. Communication with Healthcare Providers: Caregivers act as liaisons between their loved ones and healthcare providers, ensuring effective communication. They ask questions, seek clarification, and convey concerns, facilitating a better understanding of the treatment plan and fostering shared decision-making.

9. Care Coordination: Caregivers coordinate various aspects of care, including scheduling medical appointments, managing multiple healthcare providers, and ensuring seamless coordination between different specialists involved in the treatment process.

10. Medical Information Management: Caregivers organize and maintain medical records, including test results, treatment plans, and medication lists. They assist in tracking symptoms, side effects, and treatment responses, providing healthcare providers with accurate and comprehensive information.

Managing Caregiver Challenges:

Caregiving during chemotherapy treatment can be demanding and emotionally taxing. Caregivers must prioritize their own well-being to effectively support their loved ones:

11. Self-Care: Caregivers must engage in self-care activities to maintain their physical and emotional well-being. This may include taking breaks, seeking respite care, practicing stress management techniques, and attending to their own healthcare needs.

12. Seeking Support: Caregivers should reach out for support from family members, friends, and support groups. Sharing experiences, concerns, and emotions with others who have gone through similar situations can provide valuable guidance and emotional relief.

13. Education and Training: Caregivers can benefit from education and training programs that provide information

## Tips for effective caregiving

Providing care for a loved one undergoing chemotherapy is a significant responsibility that requires compassion, patience, and resilience. Effective caregiving not only supports the individual's physical and emotional well-being but also promotes a positive and nurturing environment during the chemotherapy journey. This chapter presents valuable tips for effective caregiving, emphasizing the importance of self-care, communication, and practical strategies to enhance the overall caregiving experience.

Prioritize Self-Care:

Self-care is essential for caregivers to maintain their own well-being, physical health, and emotional resilience. Here are some self-care strategies to consider:

2. Set Boundaries: Establish boundaries to balance caregiving responsibilities with personal needs. Be realistic about what you can handle and seek support when necessary. It's important to avoid burnout and maintain your own health and well-being.

3. Engage in Relaxation Techniques: Practice relaxation techniques such as deep breathing exercises, meditation, or yoga to reduce stress and promote a sense of calm. Taking breaks to engage in activities you enjoy can also help rejuvenate your energy.

4. Seek Support: Reach out to family members, friends, or support groups to share your experiences, concerns, and emotions. Seek assistance when needed and accept help graciously. Remember that asking for support is not a sign of weakness but rather a recognition of your own limitations and the importance of self-care.

5. Maintain a Healthy Lifestyle: Eat well-balanced meals, exercise regularly, and get enough restful sleep. Prioritize your own health by scheduling regular check-ups and addressing any medical concerns promptly.

Foster Effective Communication:

Open and effective communication is vital for a positive caregiving experience. Clear communication ensures that both the caregiver and the individual receiving care understand each other's needs, concerns, and expectations. Consider the following communication tips:

6. Active Listening: Practice active listening by giving your full attention to the individual and validating their thoughts and emotions. Show empathy and provide reassurance when needed.

7. Encourage Expression of Feelings: Create a safe and supportive environment where the individual feels comfortable expressing their feelings, concerns, and fears. Avoid judgment and offer non-judgmental support and understanding.

8. Share Information: Keep the individual informed about the treatment plan, medications, and potential side effects. Ensure they have a clear understanding of what to expect during chemotherapy and provide them with resources for further information if desired.

9. Collaborative Decision-Making: Involve the individual in decision-making processes related to their care whenever possible. Seek their input and respect their choices and preferences, empowering them to take an active role in their own well-being.

Practical Strategies for Caregiving:

Practical strategies can enhance the caregiving experience and improve the overall well-being of both the caregiver and the individual receiving care:

10. Organize and Coordinate: Maintain a system for organizing medical records, appointment schedules, and medication management. Keep a list of important contact numbers, including healthcare providers and emergency contacts, readily accessible.

11. Attend Medical Appointments: Accompany the individual to medical appointments, take notes, and ask questions on their behalf. This ensures that important information is captured, and clarifications can be sought.

12. Supportive Environment: Create a calm and comforting environment at home by organizing the space to meet the individual's needs. Ensure they have access to comfortable clothing, a well-stocked pantry of nourishing foods, and a quiet space for rest and relaxation.

13. Assistance with Activities of Daily Living: Help the individual with activities of daily living, such as bathing, dressing, and grooming, in a manner that respects their privacy and dignity. Provide assistance with mobility, if necessary, and make necessary adaptations to the home environment to ensure safety.

Seek Information and Resources:

Stay informed and access available resources to enhance your

## Caregiver self-care and support

Caregiving during chemotherapy treatment can be both rewarding and challenging. As caregivers devote themselves to supporting their loved ones, it is essential that they also prioritize their own well-being. Practicing self-care and seeking support are crucial elements in maintaining resilience and sustaining their caregiving role. This chapter explores the significance of caregiver self-care and support, providing valuable insights and practical strategies to empower caregivers in their journey.

Understanding the Importance of Self-Care:

Self-care is not a luxury but a necessity for caregivers. Taking care of oneself enables caregivers to provide better care to their loved ones. Here are some reasons why self-care is crucial:

2. Sustaining Energy and Resilience: Caregiving can be physically and emotionally demanding. Self-care practices help replenish energy levels, reduce stress, and maintain emotional well-being. By practicing self-care, caregivers can sustain their resilience and provide quality care over the long term.

3. Enhancing Emotional Well-being: Caregiving can bring about a wide range of emotions, including stress, guilt, and anxiety. Engaging in self-care activities helps caregivers manage these emotions, promote a positive mindset, and foster emotional well-being.

4. Improving Physical Health: Neglecting personal health can lead to burnout and health issues. Prioritizing self-care through exercise, nutritious eating, and adequate rest promotes physical well-being, enabling caregivers to fulfill their responsibilities effectively.

Self-Care Strategies for Caregivers:

Caregivers can incorporate various self-care strategies into their daily routines. Here are some effective strategies to consider:

5. Set Boundaries: Establish clear boundaries to balance caregiving responsibilities with personal needs. Learn to say no when necessary and seek support from others. Recognize that taking care of yourself is not selfish but essential for your well-being and ability to provide quality care.

6. Practice Stress Management: Engage in stress-reducing activities such as deep breathing exercises, meditation, or yoga. Find what works best for you and make it a regular part of your routine. Taking breaks, engaging in hobbies, or pursuing enjoyable activities can also help reduce stress.

7. Seek Emotional Support: Reach out to family, friends, or support groups for emotional support. Connecting with others who understand your experiences can provide validation, comfort, and valuable advice. Consider joining caregiver support groups or seeking professional counseling if needed.

8. Prioritize Personal Time: Carve out regular time for yourself, even if it's just a few minutes each day. Use this time to engage in activities that bring you joy, relaxation, and a sense of fulfillment. It could be reading, listening to music, pursuing a hobby, or simply taking a walk in nature.

9. Maintain Social Connections: Nurture your social connections by spending time with friends, family, or participating in community activities. Staying connected with others can provide a sense of belonging, support, and perspective outside of the caregiving role.

Seeking Support:

Caregivers need support, both practical and emotional, to navigate the challenges they face. Here are some avenues for seeking support:

10. Communicate with Healthcare Professionals: Stay connected with the healthcare team involved in the treatment. They can provide information, guidance, and support tailored to the specific needs of caregivers. Don't hesitate to ask questions or voice concerns about caregiving responsibilities.

11. Respite Care: Seek respite care to allow for breaks and time off from caregiving responsibilities. Reach out to family members, friends, or community organizations to arrange temporary care for your loved one. This allows you to recharge and attend to your own needs.

12. Utilize Available Resources: Investigate resources available in your community, such as respite care programs, caregiver support groups, or counseling services.

Chapter Nineteen

# Navigating Healthcare Systems

When undergoing chemotherapy, patients and their caregivers often find themselves navigating complex healthcare systems. Understanding how to effectively navigate these systems is essential for receiving quality care, accessing resources, and ensuring a smooth chemotherapy journey. This chapter explores the importance of navigating healthcare systems during chemotherapy and provides valuable insights and practical strategies to empower patients and caregivers.

Understanding the Healthcare System:

Healthcare systems can vary depending on factors such as country, insurance coverage, and healthcare providers. Familiarizing oneself with the key components of the healthcare system is crucial for effective navigation:

2. Healthcare Providers: Identify the healthcare professionals involved in your chemotherapy treatment, such as oncologists, nurses, pharmacists, and support staff. Understand their roles and how to contact them for questions, concerns, or emergencies.

3. Treatment Facilities: Be aware of the treatment facilities where chemotherapy will be administered, including hospitals, clinics, or specialized cancer centers. Understand their locations, policies, and services provided.

4. Insurance Coverage: Familiarize yourself with the specifics of your insurance coverage, including co-pays, deductibles, and coverage limitations.

Understand the process for submitting claims and seeking pre-authorization for treatments and procedures.

Building Effective Communication:

Effective communication with healthcare providers is vital for receiving the best possible care. Here are some strategies to enhance communication:

5. Be Prepared: Before medical appointments, make a list of questions, concerns, and symptoms you want to discuss. Bring along any relevant medical records, test results, and a list of current medications. This helps ensure that you make the most of your time with the healthcare provider.

6. Active Listening: Pay attention to the information provided by healthcare professionals. Take notes if necessary and ask for clarifications when needed. Actively participate in conversations and ensure you understand the treatment plan, potential side effects, and any recommended lifestyle modifications.

7. Advocate for Yourself: Be an active advocate for your own health. Don't hesitate to ask questions, seek second opinions if necessary, and express your preferences and concerns. Remember, you are an essential part of the decision-making process.

8. Utilize Technology: Take advantage of digital tools, such as patient portals, to access medical records, test results, and communicate with healthcare providers. Online resources, such as reputable medical websites or patient forums, can also provide valuable information and support.

Coordination of Care:

Chemotherapy treatment often involves multiple healthcare providers, appointments, and treatments. Effective coordination of care is essential to ensure seamless treatment and minimize gaps in communication:

9. Centralize Information: Keep a record of all medical appointments, test results, treatments, and medications in one place. This helps you stay organized and enables you to provide accurate information to healthcare providers when needed.

10. Appoint a Care Coordinator: Designate a family member, friend, or caregiver as a care coordinator. This individual can help manage appointments, track medications, and communicate with healthcare providers on your behalf. This relieves some of the logistical burdens and ensures continuity of care.

11. Establish Open Communication: Encourage open communication among healthcare providers involved in your care. Request that relevant information be shared between providers to ensure a comprehensive understanding of your treatment plan.

Accessing Supportive Resources:

Chemotherapy treatment often requires accessing supportive resources and services. Consider the following strategies:

12. Social Workers: Connect with social workers who specialize in oncology. They can provide assistance with navigating the healthcare system, financial concerns, and emotional support. They can also connect you with community resources, support groups, and assistance programs.

13. Financial Assistance: Explore financial assistance programs or resources offered by government agencies, non-profit organizations, or pharmaceutical companies. These programs can help with the cost of medications, transportation, and supportive care services.

14. Support Groups: Join support groups for cancer patients and

## Working with oncologists and healthcare teams

When undergoing chemotherapy, patients rely on the expertise and guidance of their oncologists and healthcare teams. Effective collaboration with these professionals is crucial for receiving optimal care, understanding treatment options, and navigating the complexities of the chemotherapy journey. This chapter explores the importance of working with oncologists and healthcare teams, providing valuable insights and practical strategies to foster a collaborative and supportive relationship.

The Role of Oncologists and Healthcare Teams:

Oncologists and healthcare teams play a central role in chemotherapy treatment. Their expertise, knowledge, and guidance are instrumental in providing comprehensive care. Understanding their roles is essential for effective collaboration:

2. Oncologists: Oncologists are physicians who specialize in diagnosing and treating cancer. They develop personalized treatment plans, oversee chemotherapy protocols, monitor treatment response, and address any concerns or side effects. They are the primary point of contact for patients throughout the chemotherapy journey.

3. Nurses and Nurse Practitioners: Nurses and nurse practitioners work closely with oncologists, assisting in treatment administration, monitoring patient well-being, and providing education on managing side effects. They play a crucial role in delivering compassionate care and supporting patients and caregivers.

4. Pharmacists: Pharmacists specialize in medications and their interactions. They collaborate with oncologists to ensure the appropriate selection and dosing of chemotherapy drugs. Pharmacists educate patients on medication administration, potential side effects, and drug interactions.

5. Support Staff: Support staff members, such as medical assistants and administrative personnel, contribute to the smooth functioning of the healthcare team. They assist with scheduling appointments, managing medical records, and facilitating communication between patients and healthcare providers.

Building Effective Communication:

Establishing effective communication with oncologists and healthcare teams is essential for a collaborative and supportive relationship. Consider the following strategies:

6. Prepare for Appointments: Before appointments, write down any questions, concerns, or symptoms you want to discuss. Bring a notebook or use your smartphone to take notes during the appointment to ensure you remember important information.

7. Be Honest and Open: Share your complete medical history, including any previous treatments, surgeries, or medications you are taking. Be honest about your symptoms, concerns, and lifestyle habits that may impact your treatment or well-being.

8. Ask Questions: Don't hesitate to ask questions if you don't understand something. Seek clarification on treatment options, potential side effects, and expected outcomes. Remember, well-informed patients can actively participate in decision-making and better manage their care.

9. Engage in Shared Decision-Making: Collaborate with your oncologist in developing a treatment plan. Discuss the available options, risks, benefits, and potential alternatives. Ensure that your preferences and values are considered in the decision-making process.

Advocating for Your Needs:

As a patient undergoing chemotherapy, advocating for your needs is crucial. Here are some strategies to consider:

10. Be Your Own Advocate: Take an active role in your healthcare journey by advocating for your needs and expressing your preferences. Share your treatment goals, concerns, and expectations with your healthcare team. Remember, your input is valuable in tailoring your treatment plan.

11. Seek Second Opinions: If desired, seek second opinions from other oncologists to gain different perspectives on your diagnosis and treatment options. A second opinion can provide additional information and help you make informed decisions.

12. Involve Caregivers: Engage your caregivers in discussions with your healthcare team. Their presence and input can offer valuable insights, emotional support, and help with information retention.

Accessing Additional Resources:

In addition to working closely with your oncologist and healthcare team, it's essential to leverage additional resources and support:

13. Cancer Support Organizations: Seek support from reputable cancer support organizations. These organizations provide valuable resources, educational materials, support groups, and online communities where you can

## Advocating for yourself or a loved one

When facing the challenges of chemotherapy, advocating for yourself or a loved one becomes crucial for ensuring personalized care, informed decision-making, and access to the necessary resources. Advocacy empowers individuals to take an active role in their healthcare, effectively communicate their needs, and navigate the complexities of the chemotherapy journey. This chapter explores the importance of advocacy in the context of chemotherapy, providing valuable insights and practical strategies to empower individuals as they advocate for themselves or their loved ones.

Understanding the Power of Advocacy:

Advocacy is the process of actively supporting and speaking up for oneself or others to ensure that their rights, needs, and preferences are met. When it comes to chemotherapy, advocacy is essential for several reasons:

2. Personalized Care: Advocacy ensures that care is tailored to the individual's specific needs, preferences, and values. It empowers individuals to actively participate in treatment decisions and collaborate with healthcare providers to develop personalized care plans.

3. Informed Decision-Making: By advocating for access to information, individuals can make informed decisions about treatment options, potential risks, benefits, and alternatives. They can seek second opinions, ask questions, and engage in shared decision-making with their healthcare team.

4. Access to Resources: Advocacy helps individuals access the necessary resources, support services, and financial assistance programs. It ensures that they are aware of available resources and can navigate the healthcare system effectively.

Strategies for Effective Advocacy:

Effective advocacy requires knowledge, communication skills, and determination. Consider the following strategies to advocate for yourself or a loved one during chemotherapy:

5. Educate Yourself: Take the initiative to learn about the cancer diagnosis, treatment options, and potential side effects of chemotherapy. Understanding the medical terminology and being aware of the available resources empowers you to engage in informed discussions with healthcare providers.

6. Build a Support Network: Surround yourself with a network of family members, friends, and support groups who can provide emotional support and guidance. They can offer valuable insights, share experiences, and help you navigate the challenges of advocacy.

7. Effective Communication: Develop strong communication skills to effectively express your needs, concerns, and expectations. Be assertive, clear, and respectful when interacting with healthcare providers. Prepare questions in advance, actively listen, and ask for clarification when needed.

8. Document and Organize: Maintain a record of medical appointments, test results, treatment plans, and medication regimens. Keep track of symptoms, side effects, and changes in condition. Having organized information helps you communicate effectively with healthcare providers and track the progress of treatment.

9. Seek Second Opinions: Don't hesitate to seek a second opinion from another oncologist. Obtaining different perspectives can provide additional insights and confirm or challenge the proposed treatment plan. A second opinion can contribute to your decision-making process.

Collaboration with Healthcare Providers:

Collaborating with healthcare providers is essential for effective advocacy. Here's how you can foster a collaborative relationship:

10. Establish Trust: Build a trusting relationship with your healthcare team based on open communication, mutual respect, and shared deci-

sion-making. Ensure that you feel comfortable discussing your concerns, asking questions, and expressing your preferences.

11. Prepare for Appointments: Before appointments, compile a list of questions, concerns, and any changes in symptoms or side effects. Be prepared to discuss treatment options, medication adjustments, and supportive care needs. This ensures that you make the most of your time with the healthcare provider.

12. Engage in Shared Decision-Making: Actively participate in treatment decisions by discussing the available options, benefits, risks, and potential outcomes. Make sure your values, preferences, and goals are considered when developing the treatment plan.

13. Request Information and Clarification: If you come across unfamiliar terminology or have difficulty understanding the information provided

## Managing medical records and appointments

When undergoing chemotherapy, managing medical records and appointments is crucial for maintaining continuity of care, ensuring accurate information exchange, and optimizing the treatment journey. Effectively managing these aspects streamlines communication among healthcare providers, empowers patients and caregivers, and enhances the overall quality of care. This chapter explores the importance of managing medical records and appointments during chemotherapy, providing valuable insights and practical strategies for a well-organized and efficient approach.

The Significance of Managing Medical Records:

Medical records serve as a comprehensive repository of an individual's health information. Effectively managing medical records during chemotherapy offers several benefits:

2. Continuity of Care: Medical records provide a detailed account of past and ongoing treatments, test results, and other relevant information. This ensures that healthcare providers have access to the necessary information for informed decision-making and personalized care.

3. Accurate Information Exchange: Well-maintained medical records facilitate accurate and efficient information exchange among healthcare providers. This reduces the risk of miscommunication, duplication of tests or treatments, and potential errors in care.

4. Historical Perspective: Medical records offer a historical perspective on the patient's journey, allowing healthcare providers to track progress, assess treatment response, and adjust treatment plans as needed.

Strategies for Managing Medical Records:

Organizing and maintaining medical records can be overwhelming, but implementing effective strategies can help streamline the process. Consider the following strategies:

5. Centralize Information: Designate a specific location or system to store medical records. This can be a physical folder or a digital platform. Ensure that all relevant documents, including test results, treatment summaries, and medication lists, are consistently filed and updated.

6. Create a Personal Health Record: Consider maintaining a personal health record that includes essential information such as medical history, allergies, medications, and emergency contacts. This portable record can be shared with healthcare providers as needed and serve as a quick reference during medical appointments.

7. Use Technology: Leverage digital tools such as electronic health records (EHRs) or mobile applications that allow you to access and manage medical records digitally. Many healthcare systems provide patient portals, en-

abling secure access to medical information, test results, and appointment schedules.

8. Communicate Changes: Inform all healthcare providers involved in your care about any changes to medications, treatments, or medical conditions promptly. This ensures that your medical records remain accurate and up to date.

The Importance of Managing Appointments:

Managing appointments is crucial for staying on track with chemotherapy treatment, monitoring progress, and addressing any concerns. Here are some reasons why effective appointment management is essential:

9. Treatment Adherence: Regularly scheduled appointments ensure that chemotherapy treatments are administered on time, in the prescribed doses, and according to the treatment plan. This promotes treatment effectiveness and minimizes potential disruptions.

10. Monitoring and Assessment: Appointments allow healthcare providers to monitor treatment response, evaluate side effects, and make any necessary adjustments to the treatment plan. Regular check-ins help identify and address any concerns promptly.

11. Communication Opportunities: Appointments provide dedicated time for meaningful communication with healthcare providers. They offer opportunities to discuss treatment progress, ask questions, and address any new symptoms or concerns.

Strategies for Managing Appointments:

Implementing effective strategies for managing appointments can contribute to a well-organized chemotherapy journey. Consider the following strategies:

12. Maintain a Calendar: Keep a calendar or use a scheduling application to record all upcoming medical appointments, including chemotherapy sessions, follow-up visits, lab tests, and scans. Mark important dates well in advance to ensure availability and plan other activities accordingly.

13. Plan Ahead: Prepare for each appointment by compiling a list of questions, concerns, and symptoms you want to discuss. Bring along any relevant medical records, test results, or changes in medications. This ensures that you make the most of your time

Chapter Twenty

# Complementary and Alternative Medicine

Chemotherapy is a cornerstone of cancer treatment, but its side effects and impact on overall well-being can be challenging for patients. As a result, many individuals seek additional support through complementary and alternative medicine (CAM) practices. CAM encompasses various therapies and interventions that aim to enhance the effectiveness of conventional treatments, improve quality of life, and promote overall well-being. This chapter explores the role of CAM in relation to chemotherapy, providing valuable insights into different modalities and their potential benefits.

Understanding Complementary and Alternative Medicine:

Complementary and alternative medicine refers to a broad range of therapies and practices that exist outside of conventional medical approaches. While complementary medicine is used alongside conventional treatments, alternative medicine is used as a standalone approach. It is essential to note that CAM should not replace standard cancer treatments but rather be integrated into the overall care plan under the guidance of healthcare professionals.

Supportive Therapies in CAM:

2.1. Mind-Body Practices:

Mind-body practices aim to enhance the mind-body connection and promote relaxation and well-being. Some commonly used mind-body practices in the context of chemotherapy include:

2. Meditation and Mindfulness: These practices involve focusing attention and cultivating a calm and present state of mind. They can help reduce anxiety, stress, and improve overall emotional well-being.

3. Yoga: Yoga combines physical postures, breathing exercises, and meditation. It can improve flexibility, strength, and balance, as well as promote relaxation and stress reduction.

4. Tai Chi and Qigong: These ancient Chinese practices involve slow, gentle movements, and deep breathing. They enhance balance, flexibility, and mental clarity while reducing stress and anxiety.

2.2. Herbal and Nutritional Supplements:

Herbal and nutritional supplements are commonly used in CAM. However, it is crucial to consult with healthcare professionals before incorporating them into the treatment plan, as they may interact with chemotherapy drugs or affect treatment outcomes. Some commonly used supplements include:

5. Ginger: Ginger has been shown to alleviate nausea and vomiting, which are common side effects of chemotherapy.

6. Turmeric: Turmeric contains an active ingredient called curcumin, which has anti-inflammatory properties and may have potential anti-cancer effects. However, further research is needed to establish its efficacy in cancer treatment.

7. Green Tea: Green tea is rich in antioxidants and has been studied for its potential anti-cancer properties. It may also help reduce treatment-related side effects.

2.3. Acupuncture:

Acupuncture is an ancient Chinese practice that involves the insertion of thin needles into specific points on the body. It aims to restore the balance of energy flow. Acupuncture has been used to alleviate chemotherapy-induced nausea, pain, fatigue, and hot flashes.

2.4. Massage Therapy:

Massage therapy involves the manipulation of soft tissues to promote relaxation, reduce muscle tension, and relieve pain. It can help alleviate anxiety, improve sleep quality, and enhance overall well-being.

The Benefits of CAM in Chemotherapy:

The use of CAM in conjunction with chemotherapy can provide several potential benefits:

8. Symptom Management: CAM therapies, such as acupuncture and massage, can help manage treatment-related symptoms such as nausea, pain, fatigue, and anxiety. They may enhance overall comfort and well-being during the chemotherapy journey.

9. Quality of Life Improvement: Mind-body practices like meditation, yoga, and tai chi can promote relaxation, reduce stress, and improve emotional well-being. These practices empower individuals to cope with the emotional and psychological challenges associated with cancer treatment.

10. Empowerment and Active Participation: Engaging in CAM therapies can provide patients with a sense of control and empowerment over their

health. It allows them to actively participate in their treatment journey, promoting a positive mindset and greater overall satisfaction.

Integr

## The role of complementary therapies

Chemotherapy is a crucial component of cancer treatment, but it can be accompanied by various side effects and challenges. To complement conventional treatments and enhance overall well-being, many individuals turn to complementary therapies. These therapies, used in conjunction with chemotherapy, aim to alleviate symptoms, improve quality of life, and provide emotional support. This chapter explores the role of complementary therapies in relation to chemotherapy, shedding light on different modalities and their potential benefits.

Understanding Complementary Therapies:

Complementary therapies are non-conventional approaches that are used alongside conventional medical treatments to enhance overall well-being, manage side effects, and promote a sense of balance and harmony. It is important to note that complementary therapies should be integrated into the overall care plan under the guidance of healthcare professionals and should not replace standard cancer treatments.

Supportive Therapies in Complementary Medicine:

Complementary therapies encompass a wide range of practices that can be beneficial in the context of chemotherapy. Here are some commonly used modalities:

2.1. Mind-Body Practices:

Mind-body practices focus on the connection between the mind and body and aim to promote relaxation, reduce stress, and improve overall well-being. They include:

2. Meditation: Meditation involves focusing attention and redirecting thoughts to cultivate a calm and present state of mind. It can reduce anxiety, stress, and promote emotional well-being during chemotherapy.

3. Yoga: Yoga combines physical postures, breathing exercises, and meditation. It improves flexibility, strength, and balance, while also promoting relaxation, stress reduction, and mindfulness.

4. Tai Chi and Qigong: These ancient Chinese practices involve slow, gentle movements, deep breathing, and focused attention. They promote relaxation, balance, and mental clarity, while reducing stress and anxiety.

2.2. Massage Therapy:

Massage therapy involves the manipulation of soft tissues to promote relaxation, relieve muscle tension, and alleviate pain. It can enhance well-being, reduce anxiety, and improve sleep quality during chemotherapy.

2.3. Acupuncture:

Acupuncture is an ancient Chinese practice that involves the insertion of thin needles into specific points on the body. It aims to restore the flow of energy and balance in the body. Acupuncture has been used to alleviate chemotherapy-induced nausea, pain, fatigue, and hot flashes.

2.4. Music Therapy:

Music therapy involves using music and sound to promote relaxation, reduce anxiety, and enhance emotional well-being. It can be helpful in managing treatment-related stress and improving the overall quality of life during chemotherapy.

The Benefits of Complementary Therapies in Chemotherapy:

Complementary therapies, when used in conjunction with chemotherapy, offer several potential benefits:

5. Symptom Management: Many complementary therapies can help alleviate treatment-related symptoms, such as nausea, pain, fatigue, anxiety, and sleep disturbances. By addressing these symptoms, individuals experience increased comfort and better quality of life.

6. Emotional Support: Complementary therapies provide emotional support and stress reduction, which are vital components of the chemotherapy journey. Practices like meditation, yoga, and music therapy help individuals cope with the emotional and psychological challenges associated with cancer treatment.

7. Improved Quality of Life: Complementary therapies enhance overall well-being and contribute to a better quality of life during chemotherapy. They promote relaxation, reduce stress, and foster a positive mindset, enabling individuals to cope with the physical and emotional demands of treatment.

Integration into a Comprehensive Care Plan:

The integration of complementary therapies into a comprehensive care plan requires collaboration between patients, healthcare professionals, and complementary therapists. Consider the following aspects:

8. Open Communication: It is essential to have open and honest communication with healthcare providers about the use of complementary therapies. Inform them about the specific therapies you are considering to ensure coordination and avoid any potential conflicts

## Common alternative therapies

When facing the challenges of chemotherapy, individuals often seek alternative therapies as a way to complement conventional treatments, alleviate side effects, and enhance overall well-being. Alternative therapies encompass a wide range of practices that are used in lieu of traditional medical approaches. While it is important to note that alternative therapies should not replace standard cancer treatments, they can serve as valuable adjuncts in supporting patients during their chemotherapy journey. This chapter explores common alternative therapies in relation to chemotherapy, shedding light on their potential benefits and considerations.

Herbal and Botanical Medicine:

Herbal and botanical medicine involves the use of plants, plant extracts, and natural substances for medicinal purposes. Some commonly used herbs and botanicals in relation to chemotherapy include:

2. Ginger: Ginger is known for its anti-nausea properties and can help alleviate chemotherapy-induced nausea and vomiting.

3. Turmeric: Turmeric contains curcumin, a compound known for its anti-inflammatory and antioxidant properties. It may have potential anti-cancer effects and help manage treatment-related inflammation.

4. Milk Thistle: Milk thistle is commonly used to support liver health. It may assist in mitigating the liver toxicity often associated with certain chemotherapy drugs.

It is crucial to consult with healthcare professionals before incorporating herbal and botanical remedies, as they may interact with chemotherapy drugs or interfere with treatment outcomes.

Dietary Supplements:

Dietary supplements are concentrated forms of nutrients, such as vitamins, minerals, and antioxidants, that can be taken orally. Some commonly used dietary supplements in the context of chemotherapy include:

5. Vitamin C: Vitamin C is known for its antioxidant properties and immune system support. It may help reduce chemotherapy-related side effects and enhance overall well-being.

6. Omega-3 Fatty Acids: Omega-3 fatty acids, found in fish oil or flaxseed oil, have anti-inflammatory properties and may help manage treatment-related inflammation and support heart health.

7. Coenzyme Q10: Coenzyme Q10 is an antioxidant that plays a vital role in energy production within cells. It may help reduce chemotherapy-induced fatigue.

It is important to discuss the use of dietary supplements with healthcare professionals, as they may have potential interactions with chemotherapy drugs or impact treatment outcomes.

Traditional Chinese Medicine (TCM):

Traditional Chinese Medicine encompasses a range of therapies that aim to restore balance and harmony within the body. Some commonly used TCM practices in relation to chemotherapy include:

8. Acupuncture: Acupuncture involves the insertion of thin needles into specific points on the body to restore the flow of energy. It can help manage chemotherapy-induced nausea, pain, fatigue, and other side effects.

9. Chinese Herbal Medicine: Chinese herbal medicine uses a combination of herbs to address specific health concerns. It may be used to manage treatment-related symptoms and support overall well-being during chemotherapy. It is important to consult a qualified TCM practitioner

who specializes in oncology to ensure safe and effective use of herbal formulations.

Mind-Body Practices:

Mind-body practices aim to enhance the connection between the mind and body, promoting relaxation, stress reduction, and overall well-being. Some commonly used mind-body practices in relation to chemotherapy include:

10. Meditation and Mindfulness: Meditation involves focusing the mind and redirecting thoughts to achieve a state of deep relaxation and heightened awareness. It can help reduce stress, anxiety, and promote emotional well-being.

11. Yoga: Yoga combines physical postures, breathing exercises, and meditation. It can improve flexibility, strength, balance, and promote relaxation and stress reduction during chemotherapy.

12. Guided Imagery: Guided imagery uses visualization techniques to create mental images that promote relaxation and healing. It can help reduce anxiety and enhance well-being during treatment.

Massage Therapy:

Massage therapy involves the manipulation of soft tissues to promote relaxation, relieve muscle tension,

## Integrating complementary therapies with chemotherapy

Chemotherapy is a cornerstone of cancer treatment, but it often comes with a range of side effects and challenges that can impact patients' well-being. To complement conventional treatments and improve the overall experience, many individuals turn to complementary therapies. Integrating these therapies with chemotherapy can provide additional support, alleviate symptoms, and enhance overall quality of life. This chapter explores the importance of integrating complementary therapies with chemotherapy, highlighting the potential benefits and considerations for cancer patients.

Understanding Complementary Therapies:

Complementary therapies encompass a diverse range of practices that aim to enhance well-being and promote balance. They are used alongside conventional medical treatments, including chemotherapy, to provide additional support and improve overall health outcomes. It is important to note that complementary therapies should be integrated into the overall care plan in collaboration with healthcare professionals, rather than used as a substitute for standard cancer treatments.

Benefits of Integrating Complementary Therapies with Chemotherapy:

2.1. Symptom Management:

One of the significant advantages of integrating complementary therapies with chemotherapy is the potential to alleviate treatment-related symptoms. Complementary therapies such as acupuncture, massage, and herbal medicine can help manage side effects such as nausea, pain, fatigue, and anxiety. By addressing these symptoms, patients may experience improved comfort and a better quality of life throughout their treatment.

2.2. Emotional and Psychological Support:

Cancer treatment can take a toll on patients' emotional well-being. Integrating complementary therapies such as meditation, mindfulness, and counseling can provide emotional support, reduce stress, and improve coping mechanisms. These therapies promote relaxation, help patients manage anxiety and depression, and foster a positive mindset during the chemotherapy journey.

2.3. Improved Quality of Life:

Integrating complementary therapies with chemotherapy can enhance patients' overall quality of life. Practices such as yoga, tai chi, and music therapy promote physical activity, relaxation, and emotional well-being. These therapies help individuals maintain their physical function, improve sleep quality, and increase their sense of well-being and vitality.

Considerations for Integrating Complementary Therapies:

3.1. Open Communication with Healthcare Providers:

Effective integration of complementary therapies requires open and honest communication with healthcare providers. It is important to inform your medical team about your interest in using complementary therapies and discuss their potential benefits and risks. This ensures that your treatment plan is coordinated, and potential interactions or contraindications are identified.

3.2. Qualified Practitioners:

Seeking qualified practitioners who have experience in integrating complementary therapies with conventional cancer treatment is crucial. Ensure that the practitioners you choose are licensed and have a comprehensive understanding of both complementary therapies and chemotherapy. They should be willing to collaborate with your healthcare team and adhere to safety protocols.

3.3. Timing and Scheduling:

Integrating complementary therapies with chemotherapy requires careful consideration of timing and scheduling. Some therapies may be more effective during specific phases of treatment or may require adjustments based on chemotherapy cycles. Discuss with your healthcare providers and complementary therapists to develop a well-coordinated plan that optimizes the benefits of both approaches.

3.4. Safety and Potential Interactions:

While complementary therapies can offer many benefits, it is essential to be aware of potential interactions with chemotherapy drugs. Some herbal supplements or botanical remedies may interfere with treatment outcomes or cause adverse reactions. Always consult your healthcare team before incorporating any new therapies or supplements into your treatment plan to ensure safety and avoid potential conflicts.

Collaboration and Multidisciplinary Care:

Integrating complementary therapies with chemotherapy is most effective when it is part of a multidisciplinary approach to care. Collaboration among healthcare providers, including oncologists, nurses, and complementary therapists, allows for comprehensive support that addresses both the physical and emotional aspects of treatment

Chapter Twenty-One

# Chemotherapy Safety and Administration

Chemotherapy plays a crucial role in cancer treatment, helping to destroy cancer cells and prevent their spread. As a powerful medical intervention, chemotherapy requires careful administration and adherence to safety protocols to ensure its effectiveness and minimize potential risks. This chapter explores the importance of chemotherapy safety and administration, highlighting key considerations and measures taken to deliver chemotherapy safely and efficiently.

Understanding Chemotherapy:

Chemotherapy involves the use of powerful drugs to target and destroy cancer cells. It can be administered in various ways, including oral pills, injections, intravenous infusions, or topical applications. The specific drugs and treatment regimen depend on the type and stage of cancer, as well as individual patient factors.

Importance of Safety in Chemotherapy Administration:

2.1. Effective Treatment Delivery:

Ensuring safety in chemotherapy administration is vital to deliver the treatment effectively. Proper administration techniques and adherence to safety protocols help maximize the therapeutic benefits of chemotherapy and improve treatment outcomes.

2.2. Minimizing Side Effects:

Chemotherapy drugs can cause side effects, which may vary depending on the specific drugs used and individual patient factors. Adhering to safety guidelines helps minimize potential side effects and optimize patient comfort and well-being during treatment.

Safety Measures in Chemotherapy Administration:

3.1. Adequate Training and Education:

Healthcare professionals involved in chemotherapy administration undergo specialized training and education to ensure competency in handling chemotherapy drugs. They receive comprehensive instruction on proper drug handling, administration techniques, and safety protocols.

3.2. Personal Protective Equipment (PPE):

Healthcare providers who administer chemotherapy wear appropriate PPE, including gloves, gowns, masks, and protective eyewear. PPE minimizes the risk of direct exposure to chemotherapy drugs and ensures the safety of healthcare professionals.

3.3. Preparation and Mixing:

Chemotherapy drugs require careful preparation and mixing before administration. This process is performed in designated areas, such as a pharmacy or a clean room, by trained personnel following established protocols. It involves precise measurements and calculations to ensure accurate dosing.

3.4. Administration Routes and Techniques:

The choice of administration route depends on the specific chemotherapy drugs and individual patient factors. Intravenous (IV) administration is common, and healthcare professionals receive specialized training in IV catheter insertion and management to deliver chemotherapy safely. Other administration routes include oral, intramuscular, subcutaneous, and intrathecal (into the spinal fluid).

3.5. Dose Calculation and Monitoring:

Accurate dose calculation is crucial in chemotherapy administration. Healthcare providers carefully calculate the appropriate dosage based on factors such as body surface area, weight, and kidney or liver function. Regular monitoring of patients during treatment helps assess treatment response and manage any potential adverse reactions.

3.6. Safe Handling and Disposal:

Proper handling and disposal of chemotherapy drugs and related waste are essential to minimize environmental and occupational hazards. Guidelines and protocols for safe handling and disposal are strictly followed to protect healthcare providers, patients, and the environment.

Patient Education and Informed Consent:

4.1. Informed Consent:

Before starting chemotherapy, patients provide informed consent, indicating their understanding of the treatment, its potential risks and benefits, and any alternative options. Informed consent ensures that patients are actively involved in decision-making and have a clear understanding of the treatment process.

4.2. Patient Education:

Patient education plays a crucial role in chemotherapy safety. Healthcare providers offer comprehensive information about the treatment, its potential side effects, and self-care measures. Patients are educated on recognizing and reporting side effects, managing symptoms, and adhering to prescribed medications.

Monitoring and Support During Treatment:

5.1. Regular Monitoring:

During chemotherapy, patients undergo regular monitoring to assess treatment response and manage any potential side effects or complications. Blood tests,

## Chemotherapy infusion and delivery methods

Chemotherapy is a crucial component of cancer treatment, aiming to destroy cancer cells and prevent their spread. To administer chemotherapy effectively, various infusion and delivery methods are utilized. This chapter explores different chemotherapy infusion and delivery methods, highlighting their benefits and considerations in relation to cancer treatment.

Intravenous (IV) Infusion:

Intravenous infusion is one of the most common methods of delivering chemotherapy. It involves the administration of chemotherapy drugs directly into a vein using a catheter or needle. IV infusion offers several advantages:

1.1. Direct Drug Delivery:

IV infusion allows for the direct delivery of chemotherapy drugs into the bloodstream, ensuring rapid distribution throughout the body. This method enables the drugs to reach cancer cells in different areas, targeting both localized and metastatic tumors.

1.2. Flexibility and Compatibility:

IV infusion allows for the administration of multiple chemotherapy drugs in a single session. Healthcare providers can customize the treatment regimen by combining different drugs, adjusting doses, and infusing fluids to maintain hydration.

1.3. Ease of Access:

Veins in the arms, hands, or feet are commonly used for IV infusion. This accessibility makes the process convenient for patients and allows for easy monitoring during treatment.

However, IV infusion may have some limitations, including the need for frequent clinic visits, potential vein irritation or damage, and the risk of infection associated with catheter insertion.

Central Venous Catheters:

Central venous catheters are used when long-term or repeated IV chemotherapy is required. These catheters are inserted into a large central vein, such as the subclavian vein or jugular vein, and are threaded to the superior vena cava near the heart. There are several types of central venous catheters:

2.1. Implanted Port:

An implanted port is a small device placed under the skin, usually in the chest area. It consists of a reservoir attached to a catheter. The port is accessed using a special needle, allowing chemotherapy drugs to be infused directly into the bloodstream.

2.2. Tunneled Catheter:

A tunneled catheter is inserted under the skin through a small incision and tunnelled to a central vein. The catheter exits the body through a separate incision. The exposed end of the catheter is used for chemotherapy infusion.

Central venous catheters offer several advantages:

2. Long-term Access: They provide long-term access for chemotherapy administration, reducing the need for frequent needle insertions.

3. Compatibility: Multiple drugs and fluids can be administered through the catheter, streamlining the treatment process.

4. Reduced Vein Irritation: By bypassing smaller peripheral veins, central venous catheters minimize the risk of vein irritation and damage.

However, these catheters require careful maintenance to prevent infection and require regular flushing and dressing changes.

Oral Chemotherapy:

Oral chemotherapy involves taking chemotherapy drugs in pill, capsule, or liquid form. This method offers convenience and flexibility, allowing patients to take their medication at home. Benefits of oral chemotherapy include:

3.1. Independence and Convenience:

Oral chemotherapy enables patients to take their medication in the comfort of their own homes, eliminating the need for frequent hospital visits. This method allows patients to maintain their daily routines and may reduce associated costs.

3.2. Non-Invasive:

Unlike IV infusion, oral chemotherapy does not require needles or catheters, making it a more comfortable option for some patients.

However, there are considerations for oral chemotherapy:

5. Adherence: Oral chemotherapy requires strict adherence to the prescribed schedule and dosage. Patients must closely follow instructions and communicate with their healthcare team to ensure optimal treatment outcomes.

6. Absorption: The absorption of oral chemotherapy drugs can be influenced by factors such as food, other medications

## Safety precautions and guidelines

Chemotherapy is a powerful treatment modality used to combat cancer. While it is highly effective, it also carries potential risks and side effects. To ensure patient safety and minimize potential complications, specific safety precautions and guidelines are implemented throughout the chemotherapy process. This chapter explores the importance of safety precautions and guidelines in chemotherapy administration, highlighting their significance in promoting patient well-being.

Proper Training and Education:

Healthcare professionals involved in chemotherapy administration undergo specialized training and education to ensure their competence in handling chemotherapy drugs. This includes comprehensive instruction on safe handling, administration techniques, and adherence to safety protocols. Regular updates and continuing education help healthcare providers stay updated with the latest safety guidelines and best practices.

Personal Protective Equipment (PPE):

Personal protective equipment plays a vital role in chemotherapy safety. Healthcare providers who handle chemotherapy drugs or come into contact with patients receiving chemotherapy wear appropriate PPE, including gloves, gowns, masks, and protective eyewear. PPE minimizes the risk of direct exposure to chemotherapy drugs and ensures the safety of healthcare professionals.

Safe Handling and Preparation of Chemotherapy Drugs:

Chemotherapy drugs are potent medications that require proper handling and preparation to minimize the risk of exposure and ensure accurate dosing. Safety measures include:

3.1. Dedicated Preparation Areas:

Chemotherapy drugs are prepared in designated areas, such as a pharmacy or a clean room, by trained personnel following established protocols. These areas are equipped with proper ventilation systems, safety cabinets, and spill containment measures to minimize exposure and contamination.

3.2. Use of Safety Devices:

Safety devices such as closed-system drug transfer devices (CSTDs) are used during the preparation and administration of chemotherapy drugs. CSTDs help prevent drug leakage, aerosol formation, and accidental exposure, reducing the risk to healthcare providers and patients.

3.3. Double-Checking Procedures:

Double-checking procedures are employed to ensure accuracy and minimize medication errors. Healthcare professionals verify the correct drug, dose, and patient information before preparing and administering chemotherapy. This double-checking process helps prevent dosing errors and ensures patient safety.

Safe Administration Practices:

Proper administration practices are essential to minimize the risk of complications and ensure the effective delivery of chemotherapy. Some key considerations include:

4.1. Appropriate Vascular Access:

Choosing the appropriate vascular access is crucial for safe chemotherapy administration. Healthcare providers carefully assess the patient's vascular health and consider factors such as the drug's vesicant properties and infusion duration. Peripheral venous access, central venous catheters, or implanted ports are selected based on individual patient needs.

4.2. Dilution and Infusion Rates:

Chemotherapy drugs are often diluted before administration to achieve the desired concentration. Dilution ensures proper drug compatibility and minimizes the risk of local tissue damage. Additionally, healthcare providers carefully monitor and control the infusion rates to prevent complications such as infusion-related reactions or fluid overload.

4.3. Adherence to Administration Guidelines:

Strict adherence to administration guidelines ensures that chemotherapy drugs are administered correctly. Healthcare providers follow specific instructions, such as the rate of administration, premedication requirements, and any special precautions for specific drugs. Adherence to these guidelines promotes patient safety and treatment efficacy.

Monitoring and Management of Side Effects:

Regular monitoring of patients during chemotherapy treatment is essential to identify and manage potential side effects or complications. Healthcare providers closely monitor vital signs, laboratory results, and patient-reported symptoms to ensure early detection and appropriate management of side effects.

5.1. Education and Patient Empowerment:

Patient education plays a vital role in chemotherapy safety. Patients are provided with comprehensive information about the potential side effects, self-care measures, and signs of complications. This empowers patients to be actively involved

## Chemotherapy at home and on the go

Traditionally, chemotherapy has been administered in hospitals or specialized clinics. However, advancements in medical technology and patient-centered care have opened up new possibilities for chemotherapy delivery. With appropriate safety measures and guidelines, chemotherapy can now be administered at home or on the go. This chapter explores the concept of chemotherapy at home and on the go, highlighting the benefits, considerations, and safety precautions associated with these alternative settings.

Chemotherapy at Home:

1.1. Convenience and Comfort:

Administering chemotherapy at home offers patients the convenience and comfort of receiving treatment in familiar surroundings. It eliminates the need for travel to a medical facility, reducing stress and enhancing overall well-being. Patients can maintain their daily routines, spend time with family, and minimize disruptions to their daily lives.

1.2. Cost Savings:

Home-based chemotherapy can result in cost savings for patients. It eliminates the need for hospital stays, transportation costs, and potentially reduces the need for caregiver support. This can significantly alleviate the financial burden associated with cancer treatment.

1.3. Enhanced Independence:

For patients who value their independence, home-based chemotherapy allows them to take an active role in their treatment. They can actively participate in self-care, manage their treatment schedule, and feel empowered in their cancer journey.

Considerations for Chemotherapy at Home:

2.1. Patient Selection:

Not all patients are suitable candidates for home-based chemotherapy. Factors such as treatment regimen complexity, the patient's physical condition, and the presence of supportive caregivers are considered when determining eligibility. The decision to administer chemotherapy at home is made collaboratively between the patient, healthcare providers, and the patient's support network.

2.2. Safety Precautions:

Ensuring safety is of paramount importance when administering chemotherapy at home. Proper training and education are provided to patients and their caregivers to ensure they understand safe handling, administration techniques, and potential risks. Healthcare professionals perform home visits to assess the home environment, provide guidance on proper disposal of medical waste, and monitor the patient's well-being.

2.3. Access to Support:

Patients receiving chemotherapy at home must have access to a reliable support system. This may include family members, friends, or professional caregivers who can assist with treatment administration, manage potential side effects, and provide emotional support. Open lines of communication between the patient, caregivers, and healthcare providers are essential for timely intervention and support.

Chemotherapy on the Go:

3.1. Portable Infusion Pumps:

Portable infusion pumps allow patients to receive chemotherapy outside of a hospital or clinic setting. These devices are lightweight, compact, and deliver medication continuously or in programmed intervals. Portable infusion pumps offer several advantages:

3.1.1. Flexibility and Mobility:

Patients can move freely and engage in daily activities while receiving chemotherapy. This flexibility allows them to maintain a sense of normalcy, continue work or school responsibilities, and pursue their hobbies and interests.

3.1.2. Reduced Clinic Visits:

Portable infusion pumps can reduce the frequency of clinic visits, especially for long-duration infusions. This saves patients' time, reduces travel costs, and minimizes the need for prolonged hospital stays.

3.1.3. Improved Quality of Life:

Receiving chemotherapy on the go allows patients to maintain their independence and freedom. They can participate in social activities, spend time with loved ones, and experience a higher quality of life during treatment.

### 3.2. Considerations for Chemotherapy on the Go:

#### 3.2.1. Patient Suitability:

Patients must meet specific criteria to receive chemotherapy on the go. Factors such as the chemotherapy regimen, treatment duration, and the patient's overall health and mobility are evaluated to determine suitability. Not all patients or chemotherapy regimens are compatible with

Chapter Twenty-Two

# Questions to Ask Your Healthcare Team

When undergoing chemotherapy, it is essential to have open communication and a strong partnership with your healthcare team. Asking questions and seeking clarifications can help you better understand your treatment, manage potential side effects, and make informed decisions. This chapter explores a range of important questions to ask your healthcare team during chemotherapy treatment, empowering you to take an active role in your care.

Treatment Planning and Options:

1.1. What type of cancer do I have, and what stage is it in?

Understanding your specific cancer type and stage helps you grasp the nature of your condition and guides treatment decisions.

1.2. What are the goals of my chemotherapy treatment?

Knowing the intended goals of chemotherapy (e.g., curative, palliative) allows you to align your expectations and make informed decisions.

1.3. What chemotherapy drugs will I receive, and how do they work?

Understanding the drugs used in your treatment and their mechanisms of action provides insights into their effectiveness and potential side effects.

1.4. Are there alternative treatment options available?

Inquiring about alternative therapies or clinical trials helps you explore additional options and make informed decisions about your treatment plan.

Treatment Administration and Logistics:

2.1. How will my chemotherapy be administered?

Understanding the administration method (e.g., IV infusion, oral medication) helps you prepare for the treatment process and manage logistical considerations.

2.2. How long will each chemotherapy session take, and how often will I receive treatment?

Knowing the duration and frequency of chemotherapy sessions allows you to plan your schedule and make necessary arrangements.

2.3. What side effects can I expect from the chemotherapy drugs, and how can they be managed?

Inquiring about potential side effects empowers you to anticipate and address them effectively. Ask about strategies for managing side effects, such as nausea, fatigue, and hair loss.

2.4. Can I take my prescribed medications or supplements during chemotherapy?

Seek clarification on the compatibility of your existing medications and supplements with chemotherapy drugs to ensure their safe and effective co-administration.

Supportive Care and Lifestyle Considerations:

3.1. Are there specific dietary guidelines or restrictions during chemotherapy?

Understanding dietary recommendations, such as foods to avoid or those that may help alleviate side effects, can support your overall well-being during treatment.

3.2. Are there any activities or lifestyle choices I should modify during chemotherapy?

Inquire about any necessary adjustments to your routine, exercise, or travel plans to ensure your safety and optimize treatment outcomes.

3.3. Are there support groups, counseling services, or resources available to help me cope with the emotional and psychological aspects of chemotherapy?

Ask about available support systems to access emotional support, connect with others going through similar experiences, and enhance your coping strategies.

Monitoring and Follow-Up:

4.1. How will my treatment response be evaluated?

Understanding the methods used to monitor treatment response (e.g., imaging scans, blood tests) enables you to track progress and make informed decisions.

4.2. What are the signs or symptoms that warrant immediate medical attention during chemotherapy?

Inquire about the red flags or adverse reactions that require immediate medical attention, allowing you to respond promptly and seek appropriate care.

4.3. How often will I have follow-up appointments, and what will they involve?

Knowing the frequency of follow-up appointments and their purpose helps you plan your ongoing care and ensures continuity in your treatment journey.

Personalized Questions:

Tailor your questions to your specific concerns, such as fertility preservation options, managing work or school obligations, or interactions with other medical conditions or medications. Your healthcare team is there to address your individual needs and provide personalized guidance.

Remember, effective communication with your healthcare team is essential for a successful chemotherapy journey.

## Preparing for consultations

Consultations with your healthcare team are crucial moments in your chemotherapy journey. These appointments provide an opportunity to gather information, address concerns, and actively participate in your treatment decisions. By adequately preparing for these consultations, you can ensure that you make the most of your time with your healthcare professionals. This chapter explores practical steps to help you prepare for chemotherapy consultations, enabling you to engage effectively and make informed decisions.

Gather Information:

1.1. Review Your Medical Records:

Familiarize yourself with your medical history, including previous test results, imaging scans, and pathology reports. Understanding your medical background allows you to ask specific questions related to your condition and treatment.

1.2. Research Your Cancer Type and Treatment Options:

Educate yourself about your specific cancer type, its characteristics, and available treatment options. Reliable sources such as reputable medical websites, patient advocacy organizations, or books can provide valuable information. However, always discuss the information you find with your healthcare team for accurate interpretation and guidance.

1.3. Prepare a List of Questions:

Compile a list of questions you have about your cancer, treatment options, potential side effects, and any concerns or uncertainties you may have. Writing down your questions beforehand ensures that you address all your concerns during the consultation.

Take a Supportive Companion:

Consider bringing a family member, friend, or caregiver to your consultation. Having someone you trust with you can provide emotional support and help you remember the details discussed during the appointment. They can also ask additional questions or take notes on your behalf.

Organize Your Documents:

3.1. Bring Relevant Medical Documents:

Collect and bring any relevant medical documents, such as previous test results, imaging reports, or biopsy results. Having these documents available during the consultation can provide valuable context and aid in treatment planning.

3.2. Maintain a Medication List:

Create a comprehensive list of all the medications, supplements, or herbal remedies you are currently taking. Include their names, dosages, and frequencies. This information is crucial for your healthcare team to assess potential drug interactions and ensure the safe administration of chemotherapy.

Track Symptoms and Concerns:

Keep a record of any symptoms, side effects, or concerns you experience between appointments. Note the date, severity, and duration of symptoms. This record will help you provide accurate and detailed information to your healthcare team, enabling them to address your specific issues effectively.

Establish Clear Goals and Preferences:

Reflect on your personal goals and preferences for your treatment journey. Consider factors such as quality of life, treatment outcomes, and potential side effects. By articulating your goals and preferences, you can have a more meaningful discussion with your healthcare team and align your treatment plan accordingly.

Be Open and Honest:

Be open and honest with your healthcare team about your medical history, lifestyle, and any concerns or fears you may have. Clear communication helps your healthcare providers understand your needs better and tailor the treatment plan accordingly.

Take Notes:

During the consultation, take notes to capture important information and recommendations from your healthcare team. Note any instructions, treatment options discussed, or potential side effects to refer back to later. These notes will serve as a valuable resource and aid in decision-making.

Clarify and Seek Further Information:

If you don't understand something or need more information, don't hesitate to ask for clarification. Seek explanations in simple terms to ensure a clear understanding of complex medical concepts. Your healthcare team is there to support you and provide the information you need to make informed decisions.

Follow-Up and Action Plan:

Before leaving the consultation, ensure that you have a clear understanding of the next steps and the action plan moving forward. Clarify follow-up appointments, tests, or treatments that need to be

## Important questions to ask

When navigating the complexities of chemotherapy, it's crucial to ask relevant and insightful questions during consultations with your healthcare team. By doing so, you can gain a deeper understanding of your treatment, address concerns, and actively participate in decision-making. This chapter explores a range of important questions to ask during chemotherapy discussions, enabling you to gather essential information and make informed decisions.

Treatment Plan and Options:

1.1. What are the goals of my chemotherapy treatment?

Understanding the objectives of your treatment helps you align your expectations and make informed decisions about your care.

1.2. What chemotherapy drugs will be used, and how do they work?

Gaining knowledge about the specific drugs being administered and their mechanisms of action allows you to understand how they target cancer cells.

1.3. What are the potential benefits and risks associated with this treatment?

Understanding the potential benefits and risks helps you weigh the potential outcomes and make decisions based on your individual circumstances.

1.4. Are there alternative treatment options available?

Inquiring about alternative treatments or clinical trials can provide additional options for consideration and help you make well-informed decisions.

Treatment Administration and Logistics:

2.1. How will the chemotherapy be administered (intravenously, orally, etc.), and what are the associated procedures?

Understanding the administration process helps you prepare for treatment sessions and know what to expect during the procedure.

2.2. How long will each chemotherapy session last, and how many sessions will I need?

Knowing the duration and frequency of treatment sessions enables you to plan your schedule and make necessary arrangements.

2.3. Are there any dietary restrictions or recommendations during chemotherapy?

Inquiring about dietary guidelines allows you to make informed choices about your nutrition and overall well-being during treatment.

2.4. Can I continue taking my current medications or supplements while undergoing chemotherapy?

Seeking clarity on medication and supplement compatibility helps ensure the safe co-administration of different substances and minimizes potential interactions.

Potential Side Effects and Symptom Management:

3.1. What are the common side effects associated with this treatment, and how can they be managed?

Understanding potential side effects allows you to anticipate and prepare for their occurrence. Inquiring about management strategies helps you mitigate discomfort and improve your quality of life during treatment.

3.2. How should I communicate with the healthcare team regarding any side effects or concerns?

Knowing the preferred method of communication and the appropriate channels to report side effects helps you stay connected with your healthcare team and receive timely support.

3.3. Are there any signs or symptoms that require immediate medical attention?

Inquiring about specific warning signs ensures that you can recognize urgent situations and seek appropriate medical care promptly.

Supportive Care and Lifestyle Considerations:

4.1. Are there support groups, counseling services, or resources available to help me cope with the emotional and psychological aspects of chemotherapy?

Asking about available support systems can provide emotional support, guidance, and coping strategies to help you navigate the challenges of chemotherapy.

4.2. How will chemotherapy impact my daily life, including work, family, and social activities?

Understanding the potential effects of treatment on your daily life allows you to plan and make necessary adjustments to maintain a sense of normalcy.

4.3. What strategies can I implement to support my overall well-being during chemotherapy?

Inquiring about self-care practices, exercise recommendations, stress management techniques, and complementary therapies can enhance your overall well-being during treatment.

Monitoring and Follow-Up:

5.1. How will my treatment response be evaluated?

Understanding the methods used to monitor treatment response helps you gauge progress and make necessary adjustments to your care plan.

5.2. What are the scheduled follow-up appointments, and what will they involve?

Clarifying the frequency and purpose

## Communicating effectively with healthcare providers

Effective communication with your healthcare providers is essential when undergoing chemotherapy. It enables you to actively participate in your care, understand your treatment plan, and address any concerns or questions you may have. This chapter explores key strategies for communicating effectively with healthcare providers during chemotherapy, facilitating a strong and collaborative relationship.

Active Listening:

Listening attentively during consultations allows you to fully understand the information provided by your healthcare provider. Practice active listening by:

2. 1.1. Giving your full attention: Maintain eye contact, avoid distractions, and actively focus on the conversation.

3. 1.2. Asking for clarification: If you don't understand something, ask your healthcare provider to explain it further or provide examples.

4. 1.3. Taking notes: Jot down important points, instructions, or recommendations to refer back to later.

Be Prepared:

Being prepared before appointments ensures that you make the most of your time with your healthcare provider. Consider the following:

5. 2.1. Compile a list of questions: Write down any questions or concerns you have prior to the appointment, ensuring that you cover all important topics.

6. 2.2. Review your medical history: Familiarize yourself with your medical records, previous test results, or treatments, providing context for your discussions.

7. 2.3. Bring a trusted companion: Having a family member, friend, or caregiver accompany you can provide emotional support and help remember important information.

Open and Honest Communication:

Open and honest communication fosters a strong partnership with your healthcare provider. Be forthcoming about:

8. 3.1. Medical history and current medications: Provide a comprehensive overview of your medical history, including any existing conditions, surgeries, or allergies. Share a list of all medications, supplements, or herbal remedies you are taking.

9. 3.2. Symptoms and concerns: Clearly describe any symptoms, side effects, or changes you've experienced since the last appointment. Be specific about the duration, intensity, and impact on your daily life.

10. 3.3. Emotional and psychological well-being: Don't hesitate to discuss your emotional state, fears, or anxieties related to chemotherapy. Your healthcare provider can provide guidance or refer you to additional support services if needed.

Ask Relevant and Specific Questions:

Asking relevant and specific questions helps you gain a better understanding of your treatment and make informed decisions. Consider asking:

11. 4.1. Treatment options: Inquire about different treatment approaches, including their efficacy, potential side effects, and expected outcomes.

12. 4.2. Treatment timeline: Ask about the duration and frequency of chemotherapy sessions, as well as any breaks or intervals.

13. 4.3. Side effects management: Seek guidance on managing common side effects, such as nausea, fatigue, hair loss, or changes in appetite.

14. 4.4. Lifestyle considerations: Discuss any lifestyle modifications or dietary restrictions that may be necessary during chemotherapy.

15. 4.5. Support services: Inquire about available support groups, counseling services, or complementary therapies that can enhance your well-being during treatment.

Seek Explanation and Clarification:

If you encounter medical jargon or complex terms that are difficult to understand, don't hesitate to ask for clarification. Your healthcare provider should be able to explain concepts in simpler language, ensuring that you have a clear understanding of your condition and treatment.

Express Your Concerns and Preferences:

Articulate your concerns, preferences, and goals related to your treatment. Share your expectations and desired outcomes, ensuring that your healthcare provider understands your perspective and can tailor the treatment plan accordingly.

Utilize Patient Portals and Online Resources:

Take advantage of patient portals or online resources provided by your healthcare provider. These platforms often offer access to medical records, test results, educational materials, and secure messaging systems, facilitating ongoing communication between appointments.

Chapter Twenty-Three

# Chemotherapy and Exercise

When undergoing chemotherapy, it's natural to focus on medical interventions and treatments. However, incorporating regular exercise into your routine can play a significant role in managing side effects, improving well-being, and enhancing treatment outcomes. This chapter explores the impact of exercise during chemotherapy, providing an interesting and informative perspective on the topic.

Managing Side Effects:

1.1. Fatigue Management:

Chemotherapy often leads to fatigue, a common side effect. While it may seem counterintuitive, engaging in regular exercise can help combat fatigue and improve energy levels. Low-impact activities such as walking, swimming, or gentle yoga can be beneficial. Start with short sessions and gradually increase intensity and duration as tolerated.

1.2. Nausea and Digestive Issues:

Some chemotherapy drugs can cause nausea and digestive problems. Light to moderate exercise, such as gentle walking or stationary biking, can help alleviate symptoms. However, it's important to listen to your body and avoid strenuous exercise during bouts of nausea.

1.3. Neuropathy Management:

Chemotherapy-induced peripheral neuropathy (CIPN) is characterized by tingling, numbness, or pain in the hands and feet. Exercise that focuses on balance, coordination, and strength training can help manage CIPN symptoms. Examples include tai chi, resistance band exercises, and gentle stretching.

Improving Physical Well-being:

2.1. Enhancing Strength and Endurance:

Regular exercise helps improve overall strength and endurance, which can aid in daily activities and enhance quality of life. Resistance training, such as lifting light weights or using resistance bands, can help build muscle and maintain bone density.

2.2. Maintaining Healthy Body Weight:

Chemotherapy can sometimes cause weight changes, including weight loss or weight gain. Engaging in regular exercise can help manage body weight and prevent excessive weight loss or gain. Combining cardiovascular exercises, such as brisk walking or swimming, with strength training can promote a healthy body composition.

2.3. Boosting Immune Function:

Exercise has been shown to have immune-boosting effects, which can be particularly beneficial during chemotherapy. Moderate-intensity activities, like brisk walking or cycling, stimulate the immune system and help reduce the risk of infections.

Psychological Well-being:

3.1. Reducing Anxiety and Depression:

Chemotherapy can have a significant impact on mental health, leading to anxiety and depression. Exercise releases endorphins, which are natural mood boosters. Engaging in regular physical activity, such as jogging, dancing, or group exercise classes, can help reduce anxiety and improve overall mood.

3.2. Enhancing Cognitive Function:

Chemotherapy-induced cognitive impairment, commonly referred to as "chemo brain," can affect memory, attention, and concentration. Exercise has been shown to improve cognitive function and promote brain health. Activities that challenge the brain, such as dancing, playing a musical instrument, or learning a new skill, can be particularly beneficial.

3.3. Stress Reduction:

Exercise serves as a natural stress reliever, helping to reduce stress and promote relaxation. Engaging in activities like yoga, tai chi, or meditation can enhance mindfulness and contribute to overall well-being.

Safety Considerations:

4.1. Consult with Your Healthcare Team:

Before starting an exercise program during chemotherapy, it's essential to consult with your healthcare team. They can provide guidance based on your specific treatment, medical history, and current condition.

4.2. Start Slowly and Progress Gradually:

Begin with gentle exercises and gradually increase intensity and duration over time. Listen to your body and rest when needed. It's important to strike a balance between challenging yourself and not overexerting.

4.3. Choose Low-Impact Activities

## Benefits of exercise during treatment

Engaging in regular exercise during chemotherapy may seem like a daunting task, but the benefits it offers are numerous and profound. Exercise can play a vital role in managing treatment side effects, improving physical and mental well-being, and enhancing overall quality of life. This chapter explores the remarkable benefits of exercise during chemotherapy, shedding light on its positive impact on patients' lives.

Managing Treatment Side Effects:

1.1. Fatigue Management:

Fatigue is a common side effect of chemotherapy that can significantly impact daily functioning. Contrary to intuition, engaging in regular exercise can actually help combat fatigue and boost energy levels. Physical activity stimulates the production of endorphins, enhancing overall well-being and reducing fatigue. Incorporating low-impact exercises such as walking, swimming, or gentle yoga into your routine can yield substantial benefits.

1.2. Nausea and Digestive Issues:

Chemotherapy often causes nausea and digestive problems, which can hinder appetite and nutrient absorption. Exercise has been shown to alleviate these symptoms by promoting healthy digestion and reducing nausea. Light to moderate activities such as walking or stationary biking can provide relief. It is important to listen to your body and avoid strenuous exercise during episodes of nausea.

1.3. Neuropathy Management:

Chemotherapy-induced peripheral neuropathy (CIPN) is characterized by tingling, numbness, and pain in the hands and feet. Regular exercise that focuses on balance, coordination, and strength training can help manage CIPN symptoms. Activities like tai chi, resistance band exercises, and gentle stretching can improve nerve function and alleviate discomfort.

Enhancing Physical Well-being:

2.1. Building Strength and Endurance:

Chemotherapy can lead to muscle weakness and loss of stamina. Regular exercise can counteract these effects by improving muscle strength and endurance. Engaging in resistance training, such as lifting light weights or using resistance bands, promotes muscle growth and maintenance of bone density.

2.2. Maintaining Healthy Body Weight:

Chemotherapy can cause weight fluctuations, including both weight loss and weight gain. Regular exercise plays a crucial role in managing body weight, promoting a healthy body composition, and preventing excessive weight loss or gain. Combining cardiovascular exercises like brisk walking or swimming with strength training can optimize body weight and composition.

2.3. Boosting Immune Function:

Chemotherapy weakens the immune system, making patients more susceptible to infections. Regular exercise has immune-boosting effects, reducing the risk of infection and enhancing overall immune function. Moderate-intensity activities, such as brisk walking or cycling, stimulate immune cells, improving the body's ability to defend against pathogens.

Improving Psychological Well-being:

3.1. Reducing Anxiety and Depression:

Chemotherapy can take a toll on patients' mental health, leading to increased anxiety and depression. Exercise releases endorphins, neurotransmitters that promote feelings of happiness and well-being. Regular physical activity, such as jogging, dancing, or group exercise classes, can reduce anxiety and improve overall mood.

3.2. Enhancing Cognitive Function:

Chemotherapy-induced cognitive impairment, often referred to as "chemo brain," can affect memory, attention, and concentration. Exercise has been shown to improve cognitive function and promote brain health. Engaging in activities that challenge the brain, such as dancing, playing a musical instrument, or learning a new skill, can enhance cognitive abilities and offset cognitive decline.

3.3. Managing Stress and Improving Sleep:

Chemotherapy and its associated challenges can lead to heightened stress levels and disrupted sleep patterns. Exercise acts as a natural stress reliever, reducing stress hormones and promoting relaxation. Activities like yoga, tai chi, or meditation not only enhance physical well-being but also help manage stress and improve sleep quality.

Strengthen

## Safe exercise recommendations

Engaging in regular exercise during chemotherapy can be a powerful tool for managing side effects, improving physical and mental well-being, and maintaining overall health. However, it's important to approach exercise with caution and follow safe guidelines to ensure your safety and optimize the benefits. This chapter explores safe exercise recommendations during chemotherapy, providing factual and informative guidance for patients.

Consult with Your Healthcare Team:

Before starting any exercise program during chemotherapy, it is crucial to consult with your healthcare team. They can assess your individual circumstances and provide tailored recommendations based on your specific treatment, overall health, and any existing medical conditions. They will consider factors such as blood counts, treatment schedule, and potential risks associated with certain exercises.

Start Slow and Progress Gradually:

When beginning an exercise routine during chemotherapy, it's important to start slowly and gradually increase the intensity and duration of your workouts. This allows your body to adapt and reduces the risk of overexertion. Aim for short sessions of low to moderate intensity exercises and listen to your body. If you experience any unusual symptoms or discomfort, consult your healthcare team.

Choose Appropriate Types of Exercise:

3.1. Low-Impact Activities:

Opt for low-impact exercises that are gentle on the joints and muscles, reducing the risk of injury. Examples include walking, swimming, stationary biking, yoga, tai chi, and Pilates. These activities provide cardiovascular benefits, improve flexibility, and enhance overall strength.

3.2. Strength Training:

Incorporating strength training exercises into your routine can help maintain muscle mass, improve bone density, and enhance overall strength. Focus on light to moderate resistance training using weights, resistance bands, or bodyweight exercises. Perform exercises that target major muscle groups, such as squats, lunges, bicep curls, and chest presses. Start with lighter weights and gradually increase as tolerated.

3.3. Flexibility and Stretching:

Maintaining flexibility is essential during chemotherapy to prevent muscle tightness and maintain joint range of motion. Include stretching exercises in your routine to improve flexibility and reduce the risk of musculoskeletal issues. Perform gentle stretches for major muscle groups, holding each stretch for 15 to 30 seconds. Yoga or Pilates classes specifically designed for cancer patients can be beneficial.

Listen to Your Body:

4.1. Monitor Energy Levels:

Pay attention to your energy levels and adjust your exercise routine accordingly. It's normal to experience fluctuations in energy during chemotherapy. On days when you feel more fatigued, engage in lighter activities or take rest days. Be mindful not to push yourself beyond your limits.

4.2. Hydrate and Nourish:

Stay hydrated before, during, and after exercise. Chemotherapy can cause dehydration, so it's essential to drink plenty of fluids. Additionally, nourish your body with a well-balanced diet that includes adequate protein, carbohydrates, and healthy fats. Consult a registered dietitian for personalized nutritional guidance.

4.3. Recognize Warning Signs:

Be aware of warning signs during exercise, such as dizziness, shortness of breath, chest pain, extreme fatigue, or unusual pain. If you experience any of these symptoms, stop exercising and seek medical attention. These signs may indicate a need to modify your exercise routine or be evaluated by your healthcare team.

Create a Safe Environment:

5.1. Exercise with a Buddy:

Consider exercising with a friend, family member, or trained professional to ensure your safety. They can provide support, motivation, and assistance if needed. Additionally, having someone nearby can be reassuring in case of any medical emergencies.

5.2. Balance and Stability:

If you're at risk of falls or have balance issues, use appropriate aids

## Building an exercise routine

Embarking on an exercise routine during chemotherapy may seem challenging, but with careful planning and guidance, it can become an essential part of your treatment journey. Developing a structured exercise routine not only helps manage side effects but also promotes physical and mental well-being. This chapter explores the steps involved in building an exercise routine during chemotherapy, providing informative guidance and practical tips.

Consult with Your Healthcare Team:

Before starting any exercise program during chemotherapy, it is crucial to consult with your healthcare team. They are familiar with your medical history, treatment plan, and individual needs. They can provide specific recommendations and guidelines based on your condition and treatment side effects. Your healthcare team will guide you in choosing appropriate exercises, considering any limitations or precautions.

Set Realistic Goals:

When building an exercise routine, it's essential to set realistic goals that align with your current physical condition and treatment schedule. Start by identifying your overall objectives, such as improving energy levels, managing side effects, or enhancing strength and endurance. Break down these goals into smaller, achievable targets that can be accomplished within your treatment timeline.

Choose Suitable Activities:

3.1. Cardiovascular Exercises:

Cardiovascular exercises are beneficial for improving endurance, boosting cardiovascular health, and managing fatigue. Examples of low-impact cardio activities suitable during chemotherapy include brisk walking, swimming, cycling, or using a stationary bike. Begin with shorter sessions and gradually increase the duration and intensity as you build stamina.

3.2. Strength Training:

Strength training is essential for maintaining muscle mass, improving bone density, and enhancing overall strength. Use light weights, resistance bands, or bodyweight exercises to target major muscle groups. Aim for two to three strength training sessions per week, allowing for at least a day of rest between sessions. Work with a certified trainer or physical therapist who has experience working with cancer patients to ensure proper form and technique.

3.3. Flexibility and Balance Exercises:

Incorporate flexibility and balance exercises to improve joint mobility, prevent muscle tightness, and enhance stability. Gentle stretching routines, yoga, tai chi, or Pilates can promote flexibility and balance. Focus on gentle movements and modifications that accommodate your physical abilities and any physical restrictions you may have.

Start Slowly and Progress Gradually:

4.1. Warm-Up and Cool-Down:

Prioritize warm-up and cool-down exercises before and after each workout session. A warm-up prepares your body for physical activity by gradually increasing heart rate and blood flow to the muscles. It can include light cardio exercises, gentle stretching, or range-of-motion movements. Cooling down after exercise helps bring your heart rate back to normal and prevents post-exercise dizziness. Include stretching exercises during the cool-down period to improve flexibility and reduce muscle soreness.

4.2. Gradual Progression:

Begin your exercise routine with low to moderate intensity and duration, gradually increasing both as your body adapts. Listen to your body and avoid pushing yourself beyond your limits. Incrementally increase the duration of your workouts by a few minutes each week or adjust the intensity by adding light resistance or increasing the pace of your movements. Progression should be gradual to avoid overexertion and to allow for proper recovery.

Adapt to Your Energy Levels:

5.1. Listen to Your Body:

Chemotherapy affects each individual differently, and energy levels can fluctuate. Pay attention to your body's signals and adjust your exercise routine accordingly. On days when you feel more fatigued, focus on gentle exercises or opt for restorative activities like stretching or meditation.

Balance your exercise regimen with adequate rest and recovery to support your overall well-being.

5.2. Monitor Fatigue Levels:

Keep a journal or log of your energy levels and any side effects you experience.

Chapter Twenty-Four

# Mental Health and Chemotherapy

Chemotherapy is a challenging and life-altering experience that not only affects the body but also has a significant impact on mental health. The emotional toll of chemotherapy can be overwhelming, leading to anxiety, depression, and other psychological difficulties. Recognizing the importance of mental health during this journey is crucial for patients' overall well-being. This chapter explores the relationship between chemotherapy and mental health, shedding light on the challenges patients may face and providing guidance on nurturing emotional well-being.

Emotional Challenges during Chemotherapy:

1.1. Anxiety and Fear:

The diagnosis of cancer and the anticipation of chemotherapy can trigger intense anxiety and fear. The uncertainty of the treatment process, concerns about side effects, and fear of the unknown can take a toll on mental well-being. It is important to acknowledge and address these feelings and seek support to manage anxiety effectively.

1.2. Depression and Sadness:

Chemotherapy can lead to feelings of sadness, grief, and depression. The physical and emotional demands of treatment, as well as changes in appearance and lifestyle, can contribute to these emotions. Recognizing the signs of depression, such as persistent sadness, loss of interest in activities, and changes in appetite or sleep patterns, is essential. Seeking professional help is crucial for effective management.

1.3. Body Image and Self-esteem:

Chemotherapy often causes changes in appearance, such as hair loss, weight fluctuations, and skin changes. These physical changes can impact self-esteem and body image, leading to feelings of insecurity and self-consciousness. It is important to address these concerns and seek support to cope with changes in body image during treatment.

The Impact of Mental Health on Overall Well-being:

2.1. Treatment Adherence:

Maintaining good mental health is vital for treatment adherence. Psychological well-being positively affects a patient's motivation and ability to adhere to treatment protocols. When mental health is compromised, patients may experience difficulties in following medication schedules, attending appointments, and engaging in self-care practices. Prioritizing mental health can enhance treatment outcomes.

2.2. Quality of Life:

Emotional well-being significantly influences overall quality of life during chemotherapy. Patients who experience positive mental health have a better ability to cope with treatment side effects, maintain social connections, and engage in activities they enjoy. Nurturing mental health can enhance overall well-being and make the treatment journey more manageable.

2.3. Support System:

Mental health challenges can strain relationships and social support networks. Communicating openly with loved ones and healthcare providers about emotional needs can strengthen support systems. Seeking support from friends, family, support groups, or mental health professionals can provide valuable emotional support throughout the chemotherapy journey.

Strategies for Nurturing Emotional Well-being:

3.1. Open Communication:

Effective communication with healthcare providers, loved ones, and support networks is essential for maintaining emotional well-being. Expressing concerns, fears, and emotions can provide relief and foster understanding. It is important to communicate openly about mental health struggles and seek assistance when needed.

3.2. Building a Support Network:

Creating a strong support network is crucial for emotional well-being during chemotherapy. Surrounding yourself with understanding and supportive individuals can alleviate feelings of isolation and provide comfort. Participating in support groups, counseling services, or online communities specifically tailored to cancer patients can offer valuable emotional support.

3.3. Seeking Professional Help:

If emotional challenges become overwhelming, it is important to seek professional help. Mental health professionals, such as psychologists or counselors with experience in oncology, can provide guidance and support in managing anxiety, depression, and other mental health issues. They can offer therapeutic interventions tailored to the unique needs of patients undergoing chemotherapy.

3.4. Mind-Body Techniques:

Incorporating mind-body techniques into daily life

## The impact of chemotherapy on mental health

Chemotherapy, as a vital component of cancer treatment, plays a significant role in improving patients' physical health. However, it is important to recognize that chemotherapy can also have a profound impact on mental health. The emotional challenges that patients experience during treatment can be just as demanding as the physical side effects. This chapter explores the impact of chemotherapy on mental health, shedding light on the various factors that contribute to emotional distress and providing insights into nurturing emotional well-being throughout the treatment process.

Emotional Challenges during Chemotherapy:

1.1. Anxiety and Fear:

Chemotherapy often triggers feelings of anxiety and fear. The diagnosis of cancer and the anticipation of treatment can lead to uncertainty and worry about the future. Patients may have concerns about treatment outcomes, side effects, and the impact on their daily lives. It is crucial to acknowledge these emotions and seek appropriate support to manage anxiety effectively.

1.2. Depression and Mood Changes:

Chemotherapy can also contribute to depression and mood changes. The physical demands of treatment, as well as the emotional toll of coping with a serious illness, can lead to feelings of sadness, hopelessness, and a loss of interest in previously enjoyed activities. Recognizing the signs of depression, such as persistent sadness, changes in appetite or sleep patterns, and a lack of motivation, is important for timely intervention and support.

1.3. Body Image and Self-esteem:

The physical side effects of chemotherapy, such as hair loss, changes in weight, and skin issues, can significantly impact body image and self-esteem. Patients may struggle with their changed appearance and experience a loss of confidence and self-worth. Coping with these challenges and finding ways to rebuild self-esteem are essential for overall well-being.

Contributing Factors to Emotional Distress:

2.1. Treatment Side Effects:

The physical side effects of chemotherapy, such as fatigue, nausea, and pain, can contribute to emotional distress. Dealing with these symptoms on a daily basis can be physically and emotionally draining, affecting patients' mood, motivation, and overall outlook on life. It is important for healthcare providers to address these side effects and provide appropriate management strategies to mitigate their impact on mental health.

2.2. Treatment Duration and Uncertainty:

Chemotherapy is often administered over an extended period, requiring patients to cope with ongoing treatment sessions, multiple cycles, and potential treatment breaks. The uncertainty surrounding treatment outcomes and the need for ongoing monitoring can add to the emotional burden. Patients may experience a sense of loss of control and heightened anxiety about the future.

2.3. Social and Emotional Support:

The availability and quality of social and emotional support play a vital role in managing the emotional impact of chemotherapy. Patients who have strong support systems and access to understanding healthcare professionals, family members, friends, or support groups often fare better emotionally. On the other hand, a lack of support or feelings of isolation can exacerbate emotional distress.

Nurturing Emotional Well-being during Chemotherapy:

3.1. Communication and Education:

Open communication with healthcare providers is crucial in addressing emotional challenges. Patients should feel comfortable discussing their concerns, fears, and emotions, allowing healthcare professionals to provide appropriate support and resources. Additionally, being well-informed about the treatment process and potential side effects can alleviate anxiety and empower patients to actively participate in their care.

3.2. Building a Support Network:

Building a strong support network is essential for managing emotional distress during chemotherapy. Connecting with others who have gone through similar experiences can provide validation, empathy, and practical advice. Support groups, both in-person and online, can be valuable resources for patients to share their feelings and gain support from individuals who understand their unique challenges.

3.3. Seeking Professional Help:

When emotional distress becomes overwhelming, seeking

## Addressing anxiety and depression

Chemotherapy is a vital component of cancer treatment, designed to target and eliminate cancer cells. While the physical effects of chemotherapy are well-known, it is important to recognize that the treatment process can also have a significant impact on mental health. Many patients undergoing chemotherapy experience feelings of anxiety and depression, which can further affect their overall well-being. This chapter explores the challenges of anxiety and depression during chemotherapy, providing insights into their causes and offering strategies for addressing these emotional issues effectively.

The Challenges of Anxiety during Chemotherapy:

1.1. Uncertainty and Fear:

The diagnosis of cancer and the start of chemotherapy can evoke feelings of uncertainty and fear. The treatment process introduces significant changes to patients' lives, both physically and emotionally. The fear of the unknown, concerns about treatment outcomes, and the potential for side effects can all contribute to heightened anxiety levels.

1.2. Treatment-related Anxiety:

Chemotherapy sessions themselves can induce anxiety. The anticipation of treatment, the clinical environment, and the associated side effects can be distressing. Patients may develop anxiety before each session, experiencing symptoms such as increased heart rate, difficulty breathing, and restlessness.

1.3. Coping with Treatment Side Effects:

The physical side effects of chemotherapy, such as nausea, fatigue, and hair loss, can also contribute to anxiety. Patients may worry about how they will manage these side effects and how they will impact their quality of life. The fear of being unable to handle treatment-related symptoms can intensify anxiety levels.

The Impact of Depression during Chemotherapy:

2.1. Feelings of Sadness and Hopelessness:

Depression can manifest as persistent feelings of sadness, hopelessness, and a lack of interest in previously enjoyed activities. The emotional burden of chemotherapy, coupled with the physical and lifestyle changes it brings, can contribute to these feelings. Patients may struggle to find joy or meaning in their lives during treatment.

2.2. Fatigue and Loss of Energy:

Fatigue is a common side effect of chemotherapy and can significantly impact emotional well-being. Constant exhaustion and a lack of energy can make it challenging for patients to engage in daily activities or maintain a sense of normalcy. The persistent feeling of tiredness can further exacerbate depressive symptoms.

2.3. Body Image and Self-esteem:

Chemotherapy often causes changes in physical appearance, such as hair loss or weight fluctuations. These changes can affect patients' body image and self-esteem, leading to feelings of self-consciousness and diminished self-worth. Coping with these changes can contribute to depressive symptoms.

Strategies for Addressing Anxiety and Depression:

3.1. Open Communication:

One of the most important steps in addressing anxiety and depression is to openly communicate with healthcare providers, loved ones, and support networks. Sharing concerns, fears, and emotions allows others to offer support and assistance. Healthcare providers can provide guidance, offer coping strategies, or refer patients to mental health professionals when necessary.

3.2. Seeking Professional Help:

When anxiety or depression becomes overwhelming, seeking professional help is crucial. Mental health professionals, such as psychologists or counselors, can provide therapy and support tailored to the unique challenges faced by cancer patients. Therapy sessions can help patients develop coping mechanisms, address negative thought patterns, and navigate the emotional challenges of chemotherapy.

3.3. Support Groups and Peer Connections:

Participating in support groups or connecting with peers who have gone through similar experiences can provide invaluable support. Sharing feelings and experiences with others who understand can alleviate feelings of isolation and provide a sense of community. Support groups can also offer practical advice and coping strategies for managing anxiety and depression.

3.4. Mind-Body Techniques:

Practicing mindfulness, meditation, or relaxation exercises can help manage anxiety and depression.

## Mindfulness and relaxation techniques

Chemotherapy is a challenging and emotionally demanding journey for cancer patients. The physical side effects and the overall impact on well-being can often contribute to heightened anxiety, stress, and feelings of overwhelm. In such circumstances, incorporating mindfulness and relaxation techniques into the treatment process can offer valuable support and foster emotional well-being. This chapter explores the benefits of mindfulness and relaxation techniques in the context of chemotherapy and provides practical insights into incorporating these practices into daily life.

Understanding Mindfulness and Relaxation:

1.1. Mindfulness:

Mindfulness involves paying attention to the present moment with openness, curiosity, and without judgment. It is a practice that encourages individuals to cultivate awareness of their thoughts, emotions, and bodily sensations. By bringing attention to the present, mindfulness helps patients develop a greater sense of clarity, acceptance, and inner peace.

1.2. Relaxation Techniques:

Relaxation techniques encompass various practices that promote relaxation and reduce stress. These techniques can include deep breathing exercises, progressive muscle relaxation, guided imagery, and meditation. Relaxation techniques aim to calm the mind, relax the body, and promote a sense of tranquility.

Benefits of Mindfulness and Relaxation during Chemotherapy:

2.1. Reducing Anxiety and Stress:

Mindfulness and relaxation techniques have been shown to effectively reduce anxiety and stress levels. By focusing on the present moment and letting go of worries and concerns, patients can experience a sense of calm and relaxation. These practices help regulate the body's stress response, promote a state of relaxation, and alleviate anxiety associated with chemotherapy.

2.2. Enhancing Emotional Well-being:

Mindfulness and relaxation practices can enhance emotional well-being by fostering a greater sense of self-awareness and self-compassion. Patients can learn to observe their thoughts and emotions without judgment, cultivating a more positive and accepting mindset. These practices also promote emotional resilience, helping patients cope with the emotional challenges of chemotherapy.

2.3. Improving Sleep Quality:

Chemotherapy can disrupt sleep patterns, leading to fatigue and overall reduced well-being. Mindfulness and relaxation techniques can help improve sleep quality by promoting relaxation before bedtime. Deep breathing exercises and guided imagery can help patients unwind, quiet their minds, and prepare for a restful night's sleep.

2.4. Coping with Treatment Side Effects:

Mindfulness and relaxation techniques can assist patients in coping with treatment side effects. By bringing attention to the present moment, patients can develop a more accepting and compassionate attitude toward their physical discomforts. These practices can help patients manage symptoms such as pain, nausea, and fatigue more effectively.

Incorporating Mindfulness and Relaxation Techniques into Daily Life:

3.1. Mindful Breathing:

Deep breathing exercises are a simple yet effective way to incorporate mindfulness into daily life. Patients can take a few moments throughout the day to focus on their breath, inhaling deeply through the nose and exhaling slowly through the mouth. This practice can be particularly helpful during moments of stress or anxiety.

3.2. Guided Imagery and Visualization:

Guided imagery involves creating a mental picture of a peaceful or soothing place. Patients can listen to guided imagery recordings or create their own visualizations to induce a state of relaxation. This technique can be practiced during chemotherapy sessions or at home to promote relaxation and alleviate anxiety.

3.3. Meditation:

Meditation is a powerful practice that cultivates mindfulness and relaxation. Patients can set aside dedicated time each day for meditation, finding a quiet space and focusing their attention on their breath, a specific sensation, or a chosen mantra. Meditation can be adapted to suit individual preferences and can range from a few minutes to longer periods of practice.

3.4. Movement-based Practices:

Incorporating movement-based practices

Chapter Twenty-Five

# Chemotherapy and Sleep

Chemotherapy is a critical component of cancer treatment, designed to target and eradicate cancer cells. While the primary focus of chemotherapy is on fighting the disease, it is important to recognize that the treatment process can significantly impact sleep patterns. Many cancer patients experience disruptions in their sleep, which can further affect their overall well-being. This chapter explores the relationship between chemotherapy and sleep, shedding light on the factors that contribute to sleep disturbances and offering insights into strategies for nurturing restful nights during treatment.

Sleep Challenges during Chemotherapy:

1.1. Insomnia:

Insomnia, characterized by difficulty falling asleep, staying asleep, or waking up too early, is a common sleep disturbance among chemotherapy patients. The emotional stress, physical discomfort, and medication side effects associated with chemotherapy can all contribute to the development of insomnia.

1.2. Sleep Fragmentation:

Chemotherapy can disrupt the continuity of sleep, leading to frequent awakenings throughout the night. Patients may experience difficulties in maintaining deep sleep stages, resulting in fragmented and restless nights.

These interruptions can leave patients feeling fatigued and unrefreshed upon waking.

1.3. Fatigue and Daytime Sleepiness:

Despite experiencing disrupted sleep, many chemotherapy patients also report experiencing fatigue and excessive daytime sleepiness. This paradoxical combination can significantly impact patients' quality of life and daily functioning. Patients may struggle to find energy and motivation, affecting their ability to engage in normal activities.

Contributing Factors to Sleep Disturbances:

2.1. Psychological Factors:

The emotional burden of a cancer diagnosis and the stress associated with chemotherapy can contribute to sleep disturbances. Anxiety, depression, and worries about treatment outcomes can make it challenging to relax the mind and prepare for restful sleep.

2.2. Physical Side Effects:

Chemotherapy treatment can cause physical side effects that directly impact sleep. Nausea, pain, hot flashes, and night sweats can disrupt sleep patterns and make it difficult to find comfort and relaxation during the night. Frequent trips to the bathroom due to increased fluid intake can also interrupt sleep continuity.

2.3. Medication Side Effects:

Some medications used during chemotherapy can have a direct impact on sleep. Certain drugs may cause insomnia or excessive drowsiness, affecting the sleep-wake cycle. It is important for patients to discuss any sleep-related concerns with their healthcare providers to evaluate the potential role of medication side effects.

Strategies for Nurturing Restful Nights during Chemotherapy:

3.1. Sleep Hygiene:

Practicing good sleep hygiene is essential for promoting restful sleep. Establishing a consistent sleep schedule, creating a relaxing bedtime routine, and optimizing the sleep environment can significantly improve sleep quality. Patients should aim to create a sleep-conducive atmosphere by keeping the bedroom cool, dark, and quiet.

3.2. Stress Management:

Managing stress is crucial for improving sleep during chemotherapy. Engaging in stress-reducing activities such as meditation, deep breathing exercises, or guided imagery can help calm the mind and promote relaxation before bedtime. It is important to find strategies that work best for individual needs and preferences.

3.3. Physical Comfort:

Taking steps to enhance physical comfort can contribute to better sleep. Using supportive pillows, adjusting bedding to accommodate temperature fluctuations, and practicing relaxation techniques such as progressive muscle relaxation can help alleviate physical discomfort and promote more restful sleep.

3.4. Communication with Healthcare Providers:

Open communication with healthcare providers is essential in addressing sleep disturbances during chemotherapy. Patients should discuss their sleep concerns, including difficulties falling asleep, staying asleep, or daytime sleepiness, to explore potential solutions. Healthcare providers can offer guidance, suggest medication adjustments if necessary, or refer patients to sleep specialists if needed.

3.5. Sleep Aids and Medications

## Sleep disturbances during treatment

Chemotherapy is a crucial part of cancer treatment, aimed at eradicating cancer cells and promoting recovery. However, the treatment process can bring about a range of physical and emotional changes that often disrupt normal sleep patterns. Sleep disturbances during chemotherapy can have a significant impact on a patient's well-being, affecting their energy levels, mood, and overall quality of life. This chapter explores the various sleep disturbances that can arise during treatment and offers insights into strategies for nurturing restful nights amidst chemotherapy.

2. Insomnia: The Difficulty of Falling and Staying Asleep

Insomnia is a common sleep disturbance experienced by cancer patients undergoing chemotherapy. The emotional stress, physical discomfort, and treatment-related side effects can all contribute to the development of insomnia. Patients may struggle to fall asleep initially or have difficulty staying asleep throughout the night. Factors such as anxiety, pain, and medication side effects can all contribute to insomnia during treatment.

3. Sleep Fragmentation: Disruptions in Sleep Continuity

Chemotherapy can lead to sleep fragmentation, characterized by frequent awakenings throughout the night. Patients may experience difficulties maintaining deep and restorative sleep stages, leading to a restless and disrupted sleep pattern. Factors such as physical discomfort, night sweats, and increased need to use the bathroom can interrupt the continuity of sleep, leaving patients feeling fatigued and unrested.

4. Circadian Rhythm Disruptions: Altered Sleep-Wake Cycles

Chemotherapy can disrupt the body's natural circadian rhythm, the internal biological clock that regulates the sleep-wake cycle. Patients may experience changes in their sleep patterns, such as excessive daytime sleepiness or difficulty staying awake during the day. These disruptions can lead to a mismatch between the body's natural sleep-wake rhythm and the external environment, making it challenging to establish a regular sleep schedule.

Contributing Factors to Sleep Disturbances during Chemotherapy

5. 4.1. Emotional Distress: The diagnosis of cancer and the experience of undergoing chemotherapy can bring about a range of emotions, including anxiety, fear, and sadness. These emotional stressors can significantly impact sleep, making it difficult for patients to relax and fall asleep.

6. 4.2. Physical Side Effects: Chemotherapy can lead to physical side effects such as pain, nausea, hot flashes, and night sweats. These physical discomforts can disrupt sleep and make it challenging to find a comfortable sleeping position or maintain restful sleep throughout the night.

7. 4.3. Medication Side Effects: Certain medications used in chemotherapy can have sleep-related side effects. For example, corticosteroids may cause increased energy and difficulty falling asleep, while pain medications can induce drowsiness or sedation. It is essential for patients to communicate with their healthcare providers about any sleep-related concerns to explore potential solutions.

Strategies for Nurturing Restful Nights during Chemotherapy

8. 5.1. Establishing a Sleep Routine: Creating a regular sleep routine can help train the body to recognize when it is time to sleep. Going to bed and waking up at consistent times can regulate the body's internal clock and improve overall sleep quality.

9. 5.2. Creating a Sleep-Friendly Environment: Optimizing the sleep environment is crucial for promoting restful sleep. Keeping the bedroom dark, quiet, and at a comfortable temperature can create a conducive atmosphere for sleep. Additionally, using comfortable bedding and ensuring proper mattress support can enhance physical comfort.

10. 5.3. Relaxation Techniques: Engaging in relaxation techniques before bedtime can help calm the mind and prepare the body for sleep. Activities such as deep breathing exercises, progressive muscle relaxation, or guided imagery can promote relaxation and reduce anxiety.

11. 5.4. Managing Pain and Discomfort: Discussing pain management strategies with healthcare providers is essential for improving

## Tips for improving sleep quality

Sleep plays a vital role in our overall well-being, and maintaining healthy sleep patterns is especially important for cancer patients undergoing chemotherapy. However, chemotherapy can often disrupt sleep, leading to difficulties falling asleep, staying asleep, and feeling refreshed upon waking. Sleep disturbances can further impact a patient's physical and emotional well-being during treatment. This chapter explores various tips for improving sleep quality during chemotherapy, providing practical insights and strategies to nurture restful nights amidst the challenges of treatment.

Establish a Consistent Sleep Schedule:

Creating a regular sleep schedule helps regulate the body's internal clock and promotes better sleep quality. Try to go to bed and wake up at the same time each day, even on weekends. Consistency in sleep timing helps synchronize the body's sleep-wake cycle and enhances sleep efficiency.

Create a Relaxing Bedtime Routine:

Engaging in a relaxing routine before bed signals to the body that it's time to unwind and prepare for sleep. Develop a soothing bedtime ritual that includes activities such as reading a book, taking a warm bath, practicing gentle stretching or yoga, or listening to calming music. Avoid stimulating activities and electronics close to bedtime, as they can interfere with sleep.

Optimize Your Sleep Environment:

Creating a sleep-friendly environment can significantly improve sleep quality. Ensure your bedroom is dark, quiet, and cool. Use blackout curtains or an eye mask to block out light, wear earplugs or use a white noise machine to drown out noise disturbances, and maintain a comfortable room temperature conducive to sleep.

Prioritize Physical Comfort:

Physical comfort plays a crucial role in promoting restful sleep. Invest in a supportive mattress and comfortable pillows that suit your individual needs. Experiment with different sleeping positions or use extra cushions to alleviate any discomfort caused by treatment side effects. Wearing loose, breathable sleepwear can also enhance comfort during the night.

Practice Relaxation Techniques:

Engaging in relaxation techniques can help calm the mind and promote a sense of relaxation before sleep. Deep breathing exercises, progressive muscle relaxation, and guided imagery are effective techniques to reduce stress and induce a state of calmness. Consider incorporating these practices into your bedtime routine to prepare both the mind and body for sleep.

Manage Pain and Discomfort:

Chemotherapy can sometimes cause physical pain and discomfort that can interfere with sleep. Communicate openly with your healthcare team about any pain or discomfort you are experiencing. They may recommend pain management strategies, such as medications or alternative therapies, to help alleviate symptoms and improve sleep quality.

Limit Stimulants:

Certain substances can interfere with sleep, especially close to bedtime. Reduce or eliminate the consumption of stimulants such as caffeine, nicotine, and alcohol, as they can disrupt the sleep-wake cycle and affect sleep quality. Be mindful of hidden sources of caffeine, including certain medications and food products, and aim to consume them earlier in the day.

Engage in Regular Physical Activity:

Regular exercise during chemotherapy can contribute to better sleep quality. Engaging in moderate-intensity physical activity, such as walking, yoga, or gentle aerobic exercises, can help reduce anxiety, improve mood, and promote restful sleep. Consult with your healthcare team to determine the most suitable exercise regimen for your individual situation.

Manage Stress and Anxiety:

Chemotherapy can be emotionally challenging, and stress and anxiety can interfere with sleep. Practice stress management techniques, such as mindfulness meditation, deep breathing exercises, or engaging in hobbies or activities that bring you joy and relaxation. Seek support from friends, family, or a counselor to help navigate the emotional aspects of treatment.

Seek Professional Support:

If sleep disturbances persist despite implementing these strategies, consider seeking guidance from a sleep specialist. They can provide further assessment and recommend specific

## Sleep aids and medication options

Sleep disturbances are common among cancer patients undergoing chemotherapy, impacting their overall well-being and quality of life. When lifestyle modifications and other strategies alone are insufficient to improve sleep quality, sleep aids and medication options can be considered. These interventions are designed to promote restful sleep, alleviate sleep-related symptoms, and enhance the overall sleep experience during chemotherapy. This chapter explores various sleep aids and medication options available to patients, providing information on their benefits, considerations, and potential side effects.

Over-the-Counter (OTC) Sleep Aids:

OTC sleep aids are readily available without a prescription and can be useful for short-term management of sleep difficulties. They typically contain antihistamines, such as diphenhydramine or doxylamine, which have sedative effects. These medications can help individuals fall asleep faster and may provide temporary relief from insomnia. However, they may also cause drowsiness the next day and can interact with other medications, so it's important to consult with a healthcare professional before use.

Prescription Sleep Medications:

In cases where sleep disturbances persist or are more severe, prescription sleep medications may be considered. These medications are typically prescribed by a healthcare provider and include various classes of drugs with different mechanisms of action.

2. Benzodiazepines: Benzodiazepines, such as diazepam and temazepam, are central nervous system depressants that induce sedation and relaxation. They can be effective in treating insomnia, but they are generally recom-

mended for short-term use due to the risk of dependence and potential side effects, such as daytime drowsiness and impaired cognitive function.

3. Non-Benzodiazepine Hypnotics: Non-benzodiazepine hypnotics, also known as "Z-drugs," include medications such as zolpidem, zaleplon, and eszopiclone. These medications have a similar mechanism of action to benzodiazepines but are considered to have a lower risk of dependence. They are commonly prescribed for short-term treatment of insomnia and can help individuals fall asleep faster and maintain sleep throughout the night.

4. Melatonin Agonists: Melatonin agonists, such as ramelteon and tasimelteon, work by targeting the body's natural sleep-wake cycle. They mimic the effects of melatonin, a hormone involved in regulating sleep, and can help regulate sleep patterns. Melatonin agonists are generally well-tolerated and can be beneficial for individuals experiencing sleep difficulties related to circadian rhythm disruptions.

Antidepressants:

Certain classes of antidepressant medications can also be prescribed to manage sleep disturbances in cancer patients undergoing chemotherapy. These medications can help alleviate insomnia symptoms and address co-existing conditions, such as depression or anxiety, that may contribute to sleep difficulties. Some antidepressants, such as trazodone, amitriptyline, and mirtazapine, have sedating properties that can aid in promoting restful sleep.

Considerations and Potential Side Effects:

When considering sleep aids and medications, it is important to discuss potential benefits and risks with a healthcare provider. They can help determine the most appropriate medication based on an individual's specific needs and medical history. It is crucial to consider the following factors:

5. Side Effects: Sleep medications can have side effects, including drowsiness, confusion, dizziness, and impaired coordination. Some medications may also lead to tolerance or dependency if used for an extended period. Patients should be cautious about engaging in activities that require alertness, such as driving, while taking sleep aids.

6. Drug Interactions: It is essential to inform healthcare providers about all medications, including over-the-counter drugs and supplements, to avoid potential drug interactions. Certain

Chapter Twenty-Six

# Holistic Approach to Chemotherapy

Chemotherapy is a conventional cancer treatment that targets and destroys cancer cells. While it plays a crucial role in managing and eradicating cancer, it can also have various physical and emotional side effects. Recognizing the multidimensional impact of chemotherapy, a holistic approach is gaining prominence in cancer care. This approach focuses on addressing the needs of the whole person—mind, body, and spirit—to promote well-being and enhance the effectiveness of chemotherapy. This chapter explores the principles and elements of a holistic approach to chemotherapy, emphasizing the integration of complementary therapies, supportive care, and self-care practices.

Complementary Therapies:

Complementary therapies are non-conventional treatments used alongside conventional cancer therapies like chemotherapy. They aim to enhance the body's natural healing abilities, reduce treatment-related side effects, and improve overall well-being. Some common complementary therapies include:

2. Acupuncture: This ancient Chinese practice involves the insertion of thin needles into specific points on the body to promote balance and restore energy flow. Acupuncture has been shown to alleviate chemotherapy-induced nausea, pain, and fatigue.

3. Massage Therapy: Massage involves the manipulation of soft tissues to relieve muscle tension, reduce pain, and promote relaxation. It can help manage chemotherapy-related symptoms such as pain, anxiety, and depression.

4. Herbal Medicine: Herbal remedies, such as ginger for nausea or chamomile for sleep disturbances, can be used under the guidance of a qualified healthcare professional. It is essential to ensure that herbal remedies do not interfere with chemotherapy drugs.

5. Mind-Body Techniques: Practices like meditation, yoga, and tai chi focus on connecting the mind and body to promote relaxation, reduce stress, and enhance overall well-being. These techniques can help individuals cope with treatment-related anxiety and improve emotional resilience.

Supportive Care:

Supportive care, also known as palliative care, focuses on providing comprehensive support to cancer patients throughout their treatment journey. It aims to manage symptoms, alleviate distress, and enhance the overall quality of life. Key elements of supportive care during chemotherapy include:

6. Symptom Management: Healthcare providers work closely with patients to manage treatment-related side effects such as pain, nausea, fatigue, and sleep disturbances. They may prescribe medications or suggest non-pharmacological interventions to address these symptoms effectively.

7. Emotional and Psychosocial Support: Cancer diagnosis and treatment can lead to a range of emotional challenges, including anxiety, depression, and fear. Supportive care teams, including psychologists, social workers, and counselors, provide emotional support and guidance to help patients navigate the emotional aspects of chemotherapy.

8. Nutritional Support: Maintaining proper nutrition is vital during chemotherapy. Registered dietitians can work with patients to develop individualized meal plans that support overall health, manage treatment-related side effects, and optimize energy levels.

Self-Care Practices:

Self-care plays a crucial role in supporting the well-being of individuals undergoing chemotherapy. It involves adopting habits and practices that promote physical, emotional, and mental well-being. Here are some self-care practices to consider:

9. Prioritize Rest and Sleep: Restorative sleep is essential for healing and recovery. Establish a regular sleep routine, create a comfortable sleep environment, and practice relaxation techniques to promote quality sleep during chemotherapy.

10. Engage in Regular Physical Activity: Physical activity, tailored to individual capabilities, can improve energy levels, reduce treatment-related fatigue, and enhance overall well-being. Consult with healthcare providers to determine appropriate exercises during treatment.

11. Maintain a Balanced Diet: Proper nutrition is vital for supporting the body's immune system and managing treatment-related side effects. Focus on consuming a balanced diet rich in fruits, vegetables, lean proteins, and whole grains. Consult with a registered dietitian for personalized dietary recommendations.

12. Seek Emotional Support: Connect with support groups

## The role of mind-body practices

Chemotherapy is a powerful treatment that targets cancer cells, but it can also have physical and emotional side effects. To enhance the overall well-being of individuals undergoing chemotherapy, mind-body practices are gaining recognition as valuable tools. These practices acknowledge the interconnectedness of the mind and body and promote healing, relaxation, and emotional well-being. This chapter explores the role of mind-body practices in the context of chemotherapy, highlighting their benefits and their potential to support individuals on their healing journey.

Meditation:

Meditation is a practice that involves focusing attention and cultivating awareness in the present moment. It encompasses various techniques, such as mindfulness meditation, loving-kindness meditation, and guided visualization. The benefits of meditation during chemotherapy include:

2. Stress Reduction: Chemotherapy can be emotionally challenging, and meditation helps individuals manage stress, anxiety, and fear. By redirecting attention to the present moment, meditation promotes a sense of calm and relaxation.

3. Pain Management: Meditation techniques have been shown to reduce pain perception and improve pain tolerance. Individuals undergoing chemotherapy can use meditation to alleviate treatment-related pain and discomfort.

4. Emotional Resilience: Meditation cultivates emotional resilience by developing skills for observing thoughts and emotions without judgment. It allows individuals to respond to challenging emotions with greater equanimity and self-compassion.

Yoga:

Yoga is a mind-body practice that combines physical postures, breathing exercises, and meditation. It promotes strength, flexibility, and balance while also addressing emotional well-being. When integrated into chemotherapy care, yoga offers several benefits:

5. Physical Well-being: Certain yoga poses can alleviate common physical side effects of chemotherapy, such as fatigue, muscle stiffness, and joint pain. The gentle movements and stretches improve circulation and promote a sense of vitality.

6. Stress Reduction: Yoga incorporates deep breathing techniques that activate the relaxation response, reducing stress levels and promoting a sense of inner calm. Regular yoga practice can enhance emotional well-being and help individuals cope with the challenges of chemotherapy.

7. Body Awareness: Chemotherapy can sometimes create a disconnect between individuals and their bodies. Yoga fosters a sense of body awareness, allowing individuals to reconnect with their physical sensations and develop a positive relationship with their bodies.

Tai Chi:

Tai Chi is a gentle and slow-moving martial art that combines physical postures, breathing exercises, and mindfulness. It emphasizes balance, coordination, and the flow of energy within the body. The benefits of Tai Chi for individuals undergoing chemotherapy include:

8. Balance and Stability: Chemotherapy can sometimes impact balance and coordination. Tai Chi exercises improve stability and reduce the risk of falls by promoting core strength, flexibility, and body awareness.

9. Stress Reduction: The slow and deliberate movements of Tai Chi, accompanied by deep breathing, induce a state of relaxation and calmness. This helps individuals manage treatment-related stress and anxiety.

10. Quality of Life: Tai Chi has been shown to improve overall quality of life, including physical function, mental health, and emotional well-being. It can enhance energy levels, reduce fatigue, and boost mood during chemotherapy.

Guided Imagery:

Guided imagery is a practice that involves using visualizations and mental imagery to create positive experiences within the mind. It is often accompanied by calming music or a soothing voice guiding the imagery process. The benefits of guided imagery for individuals undergoing chemotherapy include:

11. Stress Reduction: Guided imagery provides a means to escape stress and anxiety by creating a mental sanctuary of peace and serenity. This practice allows individuals to shift their focus away from treatment-related concerns and into a state of relaxation.

12. Empowerment and Positivity: By visualizing positive outcomes and engaging in empowering mental imagery, individuals can cultivate a sense of optimism and resilience. Guided imagery helps to tap into the power of the mind

## Integrating holistic methods with chemotherapy

Chemotherapy is a common treatment modality for cancer, but it often comes with physical and emotional challenges. As a result, many individuals undergoing chemotherapy are exploring complementary holistic methods to enhance their well-being and support the healing process. Holistic approaches focus on the interconnectedness of the mind, body, and spirit, considering the individual as a whole. Below we will explore the integration of holistic methods with chemotherapy and their potential benefits in promoting overall health and well-being.

Nutrition and Diet:

A holistic approach to chemotherapy emphasizes the importance of a balanced and nutritious diet. Proper nutrition plays a significant role in supporting the body's immune system, optimizing energy levels, and managing treatment-related side effects. Some key considerations include:

Eating a variety of fruits and vegetables to provide essential vitamins, minerals, and antioxidants that support overall health.

Consuming lean proteins, such as fish, poultry, beans, and tofu, to aid in tissue repair and maintenance.

Incorporating whole grains and fiber-rich foods to support digestion and prevent constipation, a common side effect of chemotherapy.

Staying hydrated by drinking plenty of water and avoiding sugary beverages.

Working with a registered dietitian who specializes in oncology nutrition to develop a personalized meal plan that addresses individual needs and treatment-related side effects.

Mind-Body Practices:

Mind-body practices are an integral part of holistic approaches to health and can be beneficial during chemotherapy. These practices aim to promote relaxation, reduce stress, and enhance overall well-being. Some commonly integrated mind-body practices include:

2. Meditation: Meditation helps individuals cultivate mindfulness, reduce stress, and enhance emotional well-being. It can be as simple as focusing on the breath or engaging in guided meditation exercises.

3. Yoga: Yoga combines physical postures, breathwork, and meditation. It improves flexibility, strength, and balance, while also promoting relaxation and reducing anxiety.

4. Breathing Techniques: Deep breathing exercises, such as diaphragmatic breathing or box breathing, help activate the body's relaxation response and reduce stress.

5. Visualization and Guided Imagery: These techniques involve using the power of the mind to create positive mental images that promote relaxation, reduce pain, and enhance overall well-being.

Stress Management:

Stress management is an essential component of a holistic approach to chemotherapy. Chronic stress can negatively impact the immune system and overall health. Some strategies for managing stress include:

6. Regular Exercise: Engaging in physical activity releases endorphins, improves mood, and helps reduce stress. It can be as simple as going for a walk, practicing yoga, or participating in gentle exercise routines.

7. Relaxation Techniques: Various relaxation techniques, such as progressive muscle relaxation, deep breathing exercises, and aromatherapy, can help individuals unwind and reduce stress.

8. Support Systems: Building a strong support system of family, friends, and healthcare professionals provides emotional support and a sense of connection during challenging times.

Emotional and Psychological Support:

Chemotherapy can evoke a range of emotions, including anxiety, fear, and sadness. Integrating emotional and psychological support is essential for the holistic well-being of individuals undergoing treatment. Some avenues for emotional support include:

9. Individual or Group Counseling: Professional counseling or therapy sessions provide individuals with a safe space to express their feelings, address concerns, and develop coping strategies.

10. Support Groups: Joining support groups allows individuals to connect with others who are going through similar experiences, share information, and receive encouragement and emotional support.

11. Art Therapy and Expressive Writing: Creative outlets such as art therapy or expressive writing can help individuals process their emotions, reduce stress, and enhance self-expression.

Herbal and Nutritional Supplements:

Some individuals may choose to incorporate herbal supplements or nutritional supplements into

## Yoga, meditation, and breathwork

Chemotherapy is a challenging treatment that often takes a toll on both the physical and emotional well-being of individuals. In the face of these difficulties, mind-body practices such as yoga, meditation, and breathwork have emerged as valuable tools for supporting individuals undergoing chemotherapy. These practices are rooted in ancient traditions and offer numerous benefits that promote relaxation, reduce stress, and enhance overall well-being. Below we will explore the role of yoga, meditation, and breathwork in the context of chemotherapy and highlight their potential to support individuals on their healing journey.

Yoga:

Yoga is an ancient practice that combines physical postures, breathing techniques, meditation, and ethical principles. It emphasizes the union of the mind, body, and spirit, and offers a holistic approach to well-being. When integrated into chemotherapy care, yoga can provide the following benefits:

2. Physical Well-being: Chemotherapy can lead to various physical challenges such as fatigue, muscle weakness, and joint pain. Yoga poses (asanas) help improve strength, flexibility, and balance, promoting physical well-being and relieving treatment-related discomfort.

3. Stress Reduction: Chemotherapy often induces stress, anxiety, and fear. The combination of mindful movement, breath awareness, and meditation in yoga helps individuals relax, reduce stress levels, and cultivate a sense of calm.

4. Emotional Support: Yoga incorporates mindfulness and self-compassion, allowing individuals to become more attuned to their emotions and develop a compassionate attitude towards themselves. It can provide a safe space for individuals to process and navigate their emotions during treatment.

Meditation:

Meditation is a practice that involves focusing attention and quieting the mind. It cultivates a state of deep relaxation and heightened awareness, promoting mental clarity and emotional well-being. During chemotherapy, meditation can offer the following benefits:

5. Stress Reduction: Chemotherapy can be emotionally taxing, leading to increased stress levels. Meditation techniques, such as mindfulness meditation, help individuals cultivate present-moment awareness and develop

a non-judgmental attitude towards their thoughts and emotions. This reduces stress and fosters a sense of inner calm.

6. Emotional Regulation: Meditation enhances emotional regulation by creating space for individuals to observe their thoughts and emotions without getting caught up in them. It helps individuals develop resilience and respond to challenging emotions in a more balanced and constructive manner.

7. Cognitive Function: Chemotherapy can sometimes impact cognitive function, causing difficulties with concentration and memory. Regular meditation practice has been shown to improve cognitive function and enhance mental clarity, potentially mitigating some of the cognitive side effects of chemotherapy.

Breathwork:

Breathwork techniques involve conscious control and manipulation of the breath. They are designed to influence the body's physiological and emotional state, bringing about a sense of relaxation and well-being. Incorporating breathwork into chemotherapy care can provide the following benefits:

8. Stress and Anxiety Reduction: Deep breathing exercises, such as diaphragmatic breathing or box breathing, activate the body's relaxation response, counteracting the stress response triggered by chemotherapy. These techniques promote a sense of calm and reduce anxiety levels.

9. Energy Enhancement: Chemotherapy can cause fatigue and decreased energy levels. Certain breathwork techniques, such as Kapalabhati (skull-shining breath) or energizing breathwork, can help invigorate the body and increase energy levels, providing a natural boost during treatment.

10. Emotional Balance: Breathwork connects the mind and body, facilitating emotional regulation. By consciously altering the breath, individuals can influence their emotional state, promoting a sense of balance and inner harmony.

It is important to note that mind-body practices should be approached with caution and under the guidance of trained instructors, particularly for individuals undergoing chemotherapy. Healthcare professionals can provide recommendations on appropriate modifications and

Chapter Twenty-Seven

# Chemotherapy and Dental Health

Chemotherapy is a powerful treatment that can have significant effects on various aspects of a person's health, including dental health. The medications used in chemotherapy can cause changes in the mouth, teeth, and gums, making it crucial for individuals undergoing treatment to pay close attention to their oral well-being. Below we will explore the impact of chemotherapy on dental health and provide practical tips for maintaining oral hygiene during treatment.

Oral Side Effects of Chemotherapy:

Chemotherapy drugs can have several effects on oral health, including:

2. Mouth Sores: Chemotherapy can cause the development of painful mouth sores, also known as oral mucositis. These sores can make eating and speaking difficult, leading to discomfort and decreased quality of life.

3. Infection: Chemotherapy weakens the immune system, making individuals more susceptible to infections, including oral infections such as thrush (a fungal infection) or viral infections.

4. Dry Mouth: Some chemotherapy drugs can reduce saliva production, leading to dry mouth. Saliva plays a crucial role in maintaining oral health by neutralizing acids, preventing tooth decay, and promoting healthy gums.

5. Taste Changes: Chemotherapy can alter a person's sense of taste, making certain foods taste different or unappealing.

Tips for Maintaining Dental Health during Chemotherapy:

Although chemotherapy can pose challenges to dental health, there are steps individuals can take to minimize complications and maintain oral well-being:

6. Good Oral Hygiene: Brushing the teeth at least twice a day with a soft-bristle toothbrush and fluoride toothpaste is essential. It is also important to floss daily to remove plaque and food particles from between the teeth.

7. Regular Dental Check-ups: Before starting chemotherapy, it is advisable to visit a dentist for a thorough examination and dental cleaning. Inform the dentist about your treatment plans so they can provide appropriate care and monitor any potential side effects.

8. Gentle Oral Care: During chemotherapy, it is important to be gentle with oral care to avoid causing further irritation. Use a soft-bristle toothbrush and avoid harsh or abrasive mouthwashes. Rinse the mouth with a solution of warm water and salt to help alleviate mouth sores.

9. Moisturize the Mouth: If dry mouth is a side effect of chemotherapy, sip water frequently, use artificial saliva products, or try sugar-free gum or lozenges to stimulate saliva production. Avoid alcohol-based mouthwashes, which can further dry out the mouth.

10. Manage Mouth Sores: If mouth sores develop, avoid spicy, acidic, or rough foods that can further irritate the area. Use over-the-counter oral pain relievers or topical numbing gels recommended by your healthcare team. Additionally, ask your healthcare provider about oral rinses or medications that may help manage mouth sores.

11. Proper Nutrition: Eating a well-balanced diet is crucial for maintaining overall health during chemotherapy. Opt for soft, nutritious foods that are easy to chew and swallow. Consider consulting with a registered dietitian who specializes in oncology nutrition for personalized dietary recommendations.

12. Communication with Healthcare Providers: Inform your healthcare team about any oral symptoms or concerns you may have. They can provide guidance, prescribe appropriate medications, and refer you to a dental specialist if necessary.

13. Dental Prophylaxis: Depending on the individual's health status and treatment plan, dental prophylaxis (cleaning) may be recommended before chemotherapy treatment. This helps remove plaque and reduces the risk of infection.

Dental Care After Chemotherapy:

After completing chemotherapy, it is important to continue prioritizing oral health. Consider the following steps:

14. Follow-up Dental Visit: Schedule a follow-up dental visit to assess any changes in dental health and address any lingering issues.

Oral Health Maintenance

## Oral side effects of chemotherapy

Chemotherapy is a powerful treatment used to combat cancer, but it can also have significant side effects on various parts of the body, including the mouth. The medications used in chemotherapy can cause oral side effects that range from minor discomfort to more severe complications. It is crucial for individuals undergoing chemotherapy to be aware of these potential side effects and take appropriate measures to manage their oral health. Below we will explore the oral side effects of chemotherapy and provide practical tips for addressing and minimizing their impact.

Mucositis:

One of the most common oral side effects of chemotherapy is mucositis, which refers to inflammation and ulceration of the mucous membranes in the mouth. The lining of the mouth becomes red, swollen, and painful, making it difficult to eat, drink, and speak. Mucositis can significantly affect an individual's quality of life during treatment. To manage mucositis, consider the following tips:

2. Maintain Good Oral Hygiene: Despite the discomfort, it is important to continue practicing good oral hygiene. Gently brush your teeth with a soft-bristle toothbrush and use a mild, non-irritating toothpaste. Avoid aggressive brushing, which can worsen the inflammation.

3. Rinse with Saline Solution: Rinse your mouth several times a day with a saline solution made by dissolving a teaspoon of salt in eight ounces of warm water. This can help reduce inflammation and provide relief.

4. Avoid Irritants: Stay away from foods and beverages that may irritate the mouth, such as spicy or acidic foods, hot beverages, and alcohol. Opt for soft, bland foods that are easier to tolerate.

5. Stay Hydrated: Drink plenty of fluids to prevent dehydration and keep the mouth moist. Sipping water throughout the day can help alleviate discomfort.

6. Use Topical Analgesics: Over-the-counter oral gels or rinses containing ingredients like benzocaine or lidocaine can provide temporary pain relief. Follow the instructions provided and consult with your healthcare team if you have any concerns.

Dry Mouth:

Dry mouth, also known as xerostomia, is another common side effect of chemotherapy. The medications can reduce the production of saliva, leading to a dry, sticky feeling in the mouth. This can increase the risk of tooth decay, gum disease, and oral infections. To manage dry mouth, consider the following strategies:

7. Stay Hydrated: Drink water throughout the day to keep the mouth moist. Sipping water can also help with swallowing and speech.

8. Avoid Dehydrating Substances: Limit the consumption of caffeine, alcohol, and tobacco, as they can further dry out the mouth.

9. Use Saliva Substitutes: Artificial saliva products, available as sprays, rinses, or gels, can provide temporary relief by moistening the mouth. Consult with your healthcare team or pharmacist for recommendations.

10. Chew Sugarless Gum or Suck on Sugar-Free Candy: Chewing gum or sucking on sugar-free candy can help stimulate saliva flow. Look for products sweetened with xylitol, which can help prevent tooth decay.

11. Consider Saliva-Stimulating Medications: In some cases, your healthcare team may prescribe medications that help stimulate saliva production. Discuss this option with your healthcare provider.

Infection:

Chemotherapy can weaken the immune system, making individuals more susceptible to infections, including oral infections. Common oral infections that can occur during chemotherapy include thrush (an overgrowth of yeast) and viral infections. To prevent and manage infections, consider the following:

12. Practice Good Oral Hygiene: Maintain a thorough oral hygiene routine to minimize the risk of infections. Brush your teeth at least twice a day and floss daily.

## Dental care during treatment

When undergoing chemotherapy treatment, it is essential to pay close attention to dental care to prevent and manage potential oral complications. The medications used in chemotherapy can have significant effects on oral health, including the development of mouth sores, increased risk of infections, and changes in saliva production. Below we will explore the importance of dental care during chemotherapy and provide practical tips for maintaining oral health throughout treatment.

Preparing for Treatment:

Before starting chemotherapy, it is crucial to visit a dentist for a comprehensive dental examination and cleaning. This allows the dentist to address any existing dental issues and provide appropriate care to minimize complications during treatment. During this visit, inform your dentist about your upcoming chemotherapy treatment, as they may need to adjust their approach based on your specific needs.

Maintain Good Oral Hygiene:

During chemotherapy, it is important to maintain good oral hygiene practices to minimize the risk of oral complications. Here are some key points to consider:

2. Brushing: Brush your teeth at least twice a day using a soft-bristle toothbrush and fluoride toothpaste. Be gentle and thorough, paying attention to all areas of your mouth. If your gums are sensitive or bleeding, consult your dentist for appropriate recommendations.

3. Flossing: Floss daily to remove plaque and food particles from between your teeth. Use gentle motions and avoid being too forceful to prevent gum irritation. If flossing is challenging due to mouth sores or other complications, ask your dentist for alternative cleaning methods.

4. Mouth Rinse: Your dentist may recommend a mild mouth rinse or an antimicrobial rinse to help reduce the risk of infections. Use as directed and avoid mouth rinses that contain alcohol, as they can be drying and irritating.

Managing Mouth Sores:

Mouth sores, also known as oral mucositis, are a common side effect of chemotherapy. These painful ulcers can make it difficult to eat, drink, and maintain oral hygiene. Here are some tips for managing mouth sores:

5. Soft Diet: Stick to soft, easy-to-chew foods that are gentle on your mouth. Avoid spicy, acidic, or rough-textured foods that can further irritate the sores.

6. Rinse with Saltwater: Rinse your mouth several times a day with a solution of warm water and salt. This can help soothe the sores and promote healing. Mix a teaspoon of salt in eight ounces of warm water and swish it around your mouth for 30 seconds before spitting it out.

7. Topical Treatments: Over-the-counter oral gels or rinses containing ingredients such as benzocaine or lidocaine can provide temporary relief from pain. Apply them directly to the affected areas as directed. Consult with your healthcare team or dentist for appropriate recommendations.

8. Pain Medications: If the pain is severe, your healthcare team may prescribe pain medications or recommend over-the-counter pain relievers. Follow their instructions and dosage recommendations carefully.

Addressing Dry Mouth:

Dry mouth, or xerostomia, is a common side effect of chemotherapy. It occurs when the salivary glands do not produce enough saliva, leading to discomfort and an increased risk of tooth decay. Here are some strategies to manage dry mouth:

9. Hydration: Drink plenty of water throughout the day to keep your mouth moist. Sip water regularly and consider using a humidifier at night to add moisture to the air.

10. Sugar-Free Gum and Lozenges: Chewing sugar-free gum or sucking on sugar-free lozenges can stimulate saliva production. Look for products sweetened with xylitol, as it can help reduce the risk of tooth decay.

11. Saliva Substitutes: Artificial saliva products, available as sprays,

## Preventing oral complications

Chemotherapy is a powerful treatment that can have various side effects, including oral complications. These complications can range from mild discomfort to severe issues that impact a person's ability to eat, speak, and maintain proper oral hygiene. It is important for individuals undergoing chemotherapy to take proactive measures to prevent and minimize oral complications. Below we will explore practical strategies for preventing oral complications during chemotherapy.

Regular Dental Check-ups:

Before starting chemotherapy, it is crucial to visit a dentist for a comprehensive dental examination and cleaning. This allows the dentist to identify and address any existing oral health issues, such as cavities, gum disease, or infections. Treating these conditions before chemotherapy helps create a healthier oral environment and reduces the risk of complications during treatment.

Maintain Excellent Oral Hygiene:

Proper oral hygiene is essential in preventing oral complications during chemotherapy. Here are some key practices to follow:

2. Brushing: Brush your teeth at least twice a day using a soft-bristle toothbrush and fluoride toothpaste. Pay attention to all surfaces of your teeth, including the gumline. Be gentle yet thorough to remove plaque and food particles effectively.

3. Flossing: Floss daily to clean between your teeth and along the gumline. This helps remove plaque and debris that cannot be reached by brushing alone. Use a gentle, sliding motion and avoid being too forceful to prevent gum irritation.

4. Tongue Cleaning: Use a tongue scraper or a soft-bristle toothbrush to gently clean your tongue. This removes bacteria and debris that can contribute to bad breath and oral infections.

5. Mouth Rinse: Rinse your mouth with an antimicrobial mouthwash recommended by your dentist. This can help reduce the bacterial load in your mouth and minimize the risk of infections. Avoid alcohol-based mouth rinses, as they can be drying and further irritate the oral tissues.

Hydration and Saliva Stimulation:

Chemotherapy can cause dry mouth, also known as xerostomia, which increases the risk of dental decay and oral infections. To prevent dry mouth and promote saliva production:

6. Stay Hydrated: Drink plenty of water throughout the day to maintain proper hydration. Sip water frequently, especially during and after meals.

7. Moisturize the Mouth: Use artificial saliva products, such as oral sprays or gels, to moisten the mouth and relieve dryness. These products can be purchased over the counter or recommended by your dentist.

8. Stimulate Saliva Flow: Chew sugarless gum or suck on sugar-free candies to stimulate saliva production. Look for products sweetened with xylitol, as it helps reduce the risk of tooth decay.

Nutritional Considerations:

Proper nutrition plays a vital role in maintaining oral health during chemotherapy. Good nutrition helps support the immune system and oral tissue repair. Consider the following tips:

9. Balanced Diet: Consume a well-balanced diet rich in fruits, vegetables, lean proteins, and whole grains. This provides essential vitamins and minerals necessary for oral health.

10. Limit Sugary and Acidic Foods: Reduce your intake of sugary and acidic foods and beverages, as they can increase the risk of tooth decay and irritate oral tissues. Opt for healthier snack options, such as fresh fruits and nuts.

11. Consult a Nutritionist: If you have specific dietary concerns or restrictions, consider consulting a nutritionist who can provide guidance on maintaining a healthy diet during chemotherapy.

Oral Care During Treatment Sessions:

During chemotherapy sessions, certain precautions can help protect your oral health. Inform the medical staff about your oral hygiene routine and potential oral complications. Consider the following tips:

12. Dental Protection: Ask your healthcare team if a dental guard is recommended during chemotherapy sessions to protect your teeth from damage

Chapter Twenty-Eight

# Chemotherapy and Skin Care

Chemotherapy is a powerful treatment that can have various effects on the body, including changes to the skin. These changes may include dryness, sensitivity, rash, and increased sun sensitivity. It is essential to pay close attention to skin care during chemotherapy to maintain its health and minimize discomfort. Below we will explore the importance of skin care during chemotherapy and provide practical tips for nurturing your skin throughout treatment.

Keep the Skin Hydrated:

Chemotherapy can cause dryness and dehydration of the skin. To combat this, it is crucial to maintain adequate hydration and use moisturizers regularly. Here are some tips for keeping your skin hydrated:

2. Drink Plenty of Water: Staying well-hydrated is essential for overall skin health. Drink an adequate amount of water throughout the day to maintain hydration.

3. Moisturize Daily: Apply a gentle, fragrance-free moisturizer to your entire body, paying extra attention to areas that tend to be drier, such as elbows, knees, and feet. Choose moisturizers that are hypoallergenic and free of harsh chemicals.

4. Use a Humidifier: If you experience dryness in your home, consider using a humidifier to add moisture to the air. This can help prevent excessive drying of the skin.

Protect Your Skin from the Sun:

Chemotherapy can make your skin more sensitive to the sun's harmful rays. It is important to take extra precautions to protect your skin from sun damage. Here are some guidelines to follow:

5. Apply Sunscreen: Use a broad-spectrum sunscreen with an SPF of 30 or higher. Apply it generously to all exposed areas of your skin, even on cloudy days. Reapply every two hours or more frequently if you are sweating or swimming.

6. Seek Shade: Avoid direct sun exposure during peak hours (10 am to 4 pm) when the sun's rays are the strongest. If you need to be outside, seek shade under umbrellas, trees, or wear protective clothing.

7. Wear Protective Clothing: Cover your skin with loose-fitting, lightweight clothing that provides adequate coverage. Consider wearing a wide-brimmed hat, sunglasses, and long sleeves to further protect your skin.

8. Avoid Tanning Beds: Tanning beds emit harmful UV rays that can damage your skin. Avoid using tanning beds during chemotherapy.

Gentle Skin Care Routine:

Chemotherapy can make your skin more sensitive, so it is important to adopt a gentle skin care routine. Here are some recommendations:

9. Use Mild Cleansers: Choose mild, fragrance-free cleansers that are gentle on the skin. Avoid harsh soaps or products containing irritants such as alcohol or strong fragrances.

10. Pat Dry: After bathing or washing your face, gently pat your skin dry with a soft towel instead of rubbing it vigorously. This helps to prevent irritation and preserve moisture.

11. Avoid Hot Water: Use lukewarm water for bathing or showering instead of hot water, as hot water can strip the skin of its natural oils and exacerbate dryness.

12. Skip Irritating Products: Avoid using products that may irritate your skin, such as harsh exfoliants, astringents, or products with strong fragrances. Opt for products specifically designed for sensitive or dry skin.

Protect Nails and Cuticles:

Chemotherapy can also affect the health and appearance of your nails. Here are some tips for maintaining nail health during treatment:

13. Keep Nails Clean and Dry: Cleanse your nails gently using mild soap and water. Dry them thoroughly to prevent the growth of bacteria or fungi.

14. Protect from Injuries: Avoid activities that may cause trauma to your nails, such as biting them or using them to open packages. Wear gloves while doing household chores or

## Skin changes during treatment

Chemotherapy is a powerful and effective treatment for cancer, but it can also have significant effects on the skin. Many individuals undergoing chemotherapy experience various skin changes, which can range from mild to severe. These changes may include dryness, rash, itching, sensitivity, and discoloration. Understanding these skin changes and implementing appropriate care can help alleviate discomfort and promote overall skin health. Below we will explore the common skin changes that occur during chemotherapy and provide practical tips for caring for your skin during treatment.

Dryness and Moisturization:

Chemotherapy can cause dry skin due to the drugs' impact on oil glands and moisture levels. Dry skin can feel tight, itchy, and uncomfortable. To combat dryness, it is important to keep your skin moisturized. Here are some tips:

2. Use a Gentle Moisturizer: Choose a moisturizer specifically formulated for dry or sensitive skin. Look for products that are fragrance-free, hypoallergenic, and free from harsh chemicals. Apply the moisturizer liberally after bathing and throughout the day as needed.

3. Avoid Harsh Soaps: Use mild, fragrance-free cleansers or soap substitutes that are gentle on the skin. Harsh soaps can further strip the skin of its natural oils and worsen dryness.

4. Take Shorter Showers: Prolonged exposure to hot water can deplete the skin's moisture. Limit your shower or bath time and use lukewarm water instead of hot water.

5. Humidify Your Environment: Dry air can exacerbate skin dryness. Use a humidifier in your home to add moisture to the air and alleviate dry skin symptoms.

Increased Sensitivity:

Chemotherapy can make the skin more sensitive and prone to irritation. It is important to be gentle with your skin and avoid potential triggers. Consider the following tips:

6. Choose Gentle Fabrics: Wear soft, breathable fabrics such as cotton or silk to minimize friction and irritation on the skin. Avoid rough or scratchy materials.

7. Protect Your Skin from Sun Exposure: Chemotherapy can increase your skin's sensitivity to the sun. Wear protective clothing, such as wide-brimmed hats, long sleeves, and sunglasses. Apply a broad-spectrum sunscreen with an SPF of 30 or higher to exposed skin.

8. Avoid Irritating Products: Avoid using harsh skincare products, including exfoliants, toners, and products with strong fragrances. Opt for gentle, hypoallergenic products specifically formulated for sensitive skin.

Rash and Itching:

Some individuals may develop a rash or experience itching during chemotherapy. These symptoms can be caused by an allergic reaction or as a side effect of certain chemotherapy drugs. Here are some tips to manage rash and itching:

9. Keep the Skin Clean: Gently cleanse the affected area with mild soap and lukewarm water. Avoid hot water, as it can exacerbate itching and dry out the skin.

10. Moisturize the Skin: Apply a soothing, fragrance-free moisturizer to the affected area to help alleviate itching and provide relief.

11. Use Calming Agents: Consider using over-the-counter hydrocortisone cream or other topical creams recommended by your healthcare team to reduce inflammation and relieve itching.

12. Avoid Scratching: Although it may be tempting, avoid scratching the affected area, as it can further irritate the skin and increase the risk of infection. Use cool compresses or apply gentle pressure to alleviate itching.

Discoloration and Hyperpigmentation:

Chemotherapy can sometimes cause changes in skin color, resulting in hyperpigmentation or darkening of certain areas. These changes are usually temporary and fade over time. Here are some tips to manage skin discoloration:

13. Sun Protection: Protect your skin

## Tips for maintaining healthy skin

Chemotherapy is a potent treatment for cancer that can have various effects on the body, including the skin. The skin may become dry, sensitive, and prone to other issues during chemotherapy. It is essential to prioritize skin health and take proactive steps to maintain healthy skin throughout treatment. Below we will explore practical tips for maintaining healthy skin during chemotherapy, promoting comfort and overall well-being.

Keep the Skin Hydrated:

One of the primary concerns during chemotherapy is skin dryness. To combat dryness and maintain optimal skin health, follow these tips:

1. Hydrate from the Inside: Drink plenty of water throughout the day to keep your body hydrated. This helps moisturize the skin from within.

2. Moisturize Regularly: Apply a gentle, fragrance-free moisturizer to your skin daily. Pay particular attention to areas that tend to be drier, such as elbows, knees, and feet. Choose moisturizers that are hypoallergenic, non-comedogenic, and free of harsh chemicals.

3. Use Lukewarm Water: When bathing or showering, use lukewarm water instead of hot water. Hot water can strip the skin of its natural oils and exacerbate dryness. Also, limit your bathing time to prevent excessive drying of the skin.

Protect Your Skin from the Sun:

Chemotherapy can make your skin more susceptible to sun damage. Protecting your skin from the sun's harmful rays is crucial. Follow these guidelines:

4. Apply Sunscreen: Use a broad-spectrum sunscreen with a high SPF (at least 30) on all exposed areas of your skin, even on cloudy days. Reapply every two hours or more frequently if sweating or swimming.

5. Seek Shade: Limit your sun exposure, especially during peak hours (10 am to 4 pm). Seek shade under umbrellas, trees, or wear protective clothing, such as wide-brimmed hats and long sleeves.

6. Wear Protective Clothing: Cover your skin with lightweight, loose-fitting clothing that provides adequate coverage. Consider wearing sun-protective clothing made with special fabrics that offer additional UV protection.

Maintain a Gentle Skincare Routine:

During chemotherapy, it is important to adopt a gentle skincare routine to minimize skin irritation and sensitivity. Follow these tips:

7. Use Mild Cleansers: Opt for mild, fragrance-free cleansers or soap substitutes that are gentle on the skin. Avoid harsh soaps or products containing alcohol or strong fragrances.

8. Pat Dry: After bathing or washing your face, gently pat your skin dry with a soft towel. Avoid rubbing vigorously, as it can irritate the skin.

9. Avoid Harsh Exfoliation: Skip harsh exfoliants or scrubs during chemotherapy. Instead, use gentle methods of exfoliation, such as a soft washcloth or a mild chemical exfoliator recommended by your healthcare team.

10. Moisturize Immediately: After cleansing, apply moisturizer while your skin is still slightly damp. This helps lock in moisture and provides a protective barrier.

Be Mindful of Skin Sensitivities:

Chemotherapy can increase skin sensitivity and make it prone to reactions. Be cautious with the products you use and be mindful of potential irritants:

11. Avoid Harsh Chemicals: Stay away from skincare products that contain harsh chemicals, fragrances, or dyes. Opt for gentle, hypoallergenic products specifically designed for sensitive skin.

12. Patch Test New Products: Before using new skincare products or cosmetics, perform a patch test on a small area of your skin. This will help you determine if the product causes any adverse reactions before applying it to larger areas.

13. Consult Your Healthcare Team: If you are unsure about certain skincare products or have specific concerns, consult your healthcare team for guidance. They can

## Safe and effective skin care products

Chemotherapy is a powerful treatment for cancer that can have various effects on the skin. During this time, it is essential to take extra care of your skin and use products that are safe and effective. Chemotherapy can make the skin more sensitive and prone to dryness, irritation, and other issues. Below we will discuss safe and effective skin care products that can help you maintain healthy skin during chemotherapy.

Fragrance-Free and Gentle Cleansers:

Chemotherapy can make the skin more sensitive, so it is crucial to choose a gentle cleanser that is free from harsh chemicals and fragrances. Look for cleansers that are specifically formulated for sensitive skin or recommended by your healthcare team. Fragrance-free cleansers are less likely to cause irritation and are generally safer for chemotherapy patients.

Moisturizers for Hydration:

Chemotherapy can cause dryness and flakiness of the skin. Using a moisturizer regularly can help maintain hydration and prevent dry skin. Look for moisturizers that are hypoallergenic, fragrance-free, and formulated for sensitive skin. Ingredients like hyaluronic acid and ceramides can help lock in moisture and improve skin hydration. Apply moisturizer to damp skin after bathing or washing your face to help seal in moisture.

Sunscreen for Sun Protection:

Chemotherapy can make your skin more susceptible to sun damage, so it is crucial to protect your skin from harmful UV rays. Choose a broad-spectrum sunscreen with a sun protection factor (SPF) of at least 30. Look for sunscreen that is specifically labeled as suitable for sensitive skin. Apply sunscreen generously to all exposed areas of the skin, including the face, neck, and hands. Reapply every two hours, or more frequently if you are sweating or swimming.

Mild and Soothing Skincare Products:

Chemotherapy can cause skin sensitivity, redness, and irritation. To minimize these issues, opt for mild and soothing skincare products. Look for products that are free from harsh chemicals, dyes, and fragrances. Avoid exfoliating products or harsh scrubs during chemotherapy, as they can exacerbate skin irritation. Instead, choose gentle cleansers, toners, and serums that are specifically formulated for sensitive skin.

Lip Care Products:

Chemotherapy can cause dry and chapped lips. To keep your lips moisturized and prevent discomfort, use lip care products such as lip balms or ointments. Look for products that contain natural ingredients like beeswax, shea butter, or coconut oil. Avoid products with strong fragrances or flavors, as they may irritate the sensitive skin on your lips.

Nail Care Products:

Chemotherapy can affect the health and appearance of your nails. To minimize damage and maintain nail health, use gentle nail care products. Avoid harsh nail polishes and removers that contain chemicals like formaldehyde or toluene. Instead, opt for nail strengtheners or nourishing treatments that are specifically designed for sensitive nails.

Products for Scalp and Hair Care:

Chemotherapy can cause hair loss or changes in hair texture. If you experience hair loss, you may choose to wear a wig or a head covering. Look for soft, breathable fabrics that won't irritate your scalp. Additionally, use gentle shampoos and conditioners that are free from sulfates and other harsh ingredients. If you choose to go without a wig or head covering, use sunscreen or wear a hat to protect your scalp from the sun.

Consult with Your Healthcare Team:

It is essential to consult with your healthcare team before using any new skincare products during chemotherapy. They can provide personalized recommendations based on your specific needs and treatment plan. They can also inform you of any ingredients or products to avoid

Chapter Twenty-Nine

# Chemotherapy and Bone Health

Chemotherapy is a widely used treatment for cancer that involves the use of powerful drugs to destroy cancer cells. While chemotherapy is effective in targeting cancer cells, it can also have an impact on other parts of the body, including bone health. Below we will explore the relationship between chemotherapy and bone health, and discuss strategies for protecting and maintaining strong bones during treatment.

Understanding the Impact of Chemotherapy on Bones:

Chemotherapy drugs can affect bone health in several ways. They may interfere with the production of new bone cells, leading to decreased bone density and increased risk of fractures. Some chemotherapy drugs can also cause hormonal changes that can further weaken bones. Additionally, certain treatments, such as hormone therapy or radiation therapy, may also contribute to bone loss.

Assessing Bone Health Before Treatment:

Before starting chemotherapy, it is essential to assess your bone health through a bone density test or a DEXA scan. This test measures the density of your bones and determines your risk of fractures. The results will help your healthcare team identify any pre-existing bone conditions or factors that may increase your vulnerability to bone loss during treatment.

Calcium and Vitamin D Supplementation:

Calcium and vitamin D are crucial for maintaining strong bones. During chemotherapy, it is important to ensure that you are getting enough of these nutrients. Your healthcare team may recommend calcium and vitamin D supplements to support bone health. Calcium-rich foods such as dairy products, leafy greens, and fortified foods, along with safe sun exposure for vitamin D synthesis, can also contribute to your overall bone health.

Weight-Bearing Exercises:

Engaging in regular weight-bearing exercises can help strengthen your bones and reduce the risk of bone loss during chemotherapy. Weight-bearing exercises include activities such as walking, jogging, dancing, or lifting weights. These exercises help stimulate the production of new bone cells and promote bone density. It is important to consult with your healthcare team or a physical therapist to determine the appropriate exercise routine for your specific condition.

Avoiding Tobacco and Limiting Alcohol Intake:

Smoking and excessive alcohol consumption can have negative effects on bone health. Both tobacco and alcohol can decrease bone density and increase the risk of fractures. If you are a smoker, it is highly recommended to quit smoking. If you drink alcohol, it is important to do so in moderation or as advised by your healthcare team. Taking steps to reduce these risk factors can help protect your bones during chemotherapy.

Medications for Bone Health:

In some cases, your healthcare team may prescribe medications to support bone health during chemotherapy. These medications may include bisphosphonates, which help prevent bone loss and strengthen bones. Other medications, such as selective estrogen receptor modulators (SERMs), may be prescribed to reduce the risk of fractures. It is important to discuss the potential benefits and risks of these medications with your healthcare team.

Regular Monitoring and Follow-up:

During chemotherapy, it is crucial to have regular check-ups and follow-up appointments with your healthcare team. They will monitor your bone health and adjust your treatment plan as necessary. Regular bone density tests may be performed to assess any changes in bone density and evaluate the effectiveness of the interventions in place.

Nutrition and a Balanced Diet:

A well-balanced diet plays a significant role in maintaining bone health. Along with calcium and vitamin D, it is important to consume a variety of nutrients that support bone health, such as magnesium, phosphorus, and vitamin K. Incorporate foods like dairy products, fish, nuts, seeds, whole grains, fruits, and vegetables into your diet to ensure you are getting the necessary nutrients for bone health.

Communication with Your Healthcare Team:

Open and clear communication with your healthcare team is essential throughout your chemotherapy treatment.

## The impact of chemotherapy on bones

Chemotherapy is a powerful treatment modality used in the fight against cancer. It involves the administration of drugs that target and destroy rapidly dividing cancer cells. While chemotherapy is effective in fighting cancer, it can also have unintended effects on other parts of the body, including the skeletal system. Below we will explore the impact of chemotherapy on bones and discuss strategies for managing and maintaining bone health during treatment.

Bone Remodeling and Chemotherapy:

Bone is a dynamic tissue that undergoes constant remodeling through a process known as bone turnover. This process involves the removal of old or damaged bone tissue by specialized cells called osteoclasts and the subsequent formation of new bone tissue by osteoblasts. Chemotherapy drugs can disrupt this delicate balance, leading to alterations in bone remodeling and potentially compromising bone health.

Decreased Bone Density and Increased Fracture Risk:

One of the primary concerns associated with chemotherapy is the potential for decreased bone density and increased fracture risk. Certain chemotherapy drugs, particularly glucocorticoids and aromatase inhibitors, have been linked to bone loss and osteoporosis. The decrease in bone density can make the bones more brittle and susceptible to fractures, which can significantly impact a patient's quality of life.

Hormonal Changes and Bone Health:

Some chemotherapy drugs can disrupt the normal hormonal balance in the body, leading to further complications in bone health. For example, certain breast cancer treatments that target estrogen receptors can cause estrogen deprivation, leading to accelerated bone loss. Similarly, androgen deprivation therapy for prostate cancer can contribute to bone loss in men. These hormonal changes can exacerbate the risk of osteoporosis and fractures.

Chemotherapy-Induced Early Menopause:

Chemotherapy treatments can induce early menopause in premenopausal women, leading to a decrease in estrogen levels. Estrogen plays a crucial role in maintaining bone health, and its decline can accelerate bone loss. Women who experience early menopause due to chemotherapy may be at higher risk for osteoporosis and fractures, emphasizing the importance of proactive bone health management.

Strategies for Maintaining Bone Health during Chemotherapy:

2. a. Calcium and Vitamin D: Calcium and vitamin D are essential for bone health. Adequate calcium intake, through dietary sources or supplements, helps support bone strength and integrity. Vitamin D, obtained from sunlight exposure or supplements, aids in the absorption of calcium. Both nutrients are crucial during chemotherapy to mitigate bone loss.

3. b. Weight-Bearing Exercises: Engaging in weight-bearing exercises, such as walking, jogging, or resistance training, can help stimulate bone remodeling and promote bone density. These exercises put stress on the bones, triggering the body's natural response to strengthen and rebuild them. It is important to consult with a healthcare professional to determine the appropriate exercise regimen based on individual circumstances.

4. c. Medications for Bone Health: In some cases, healthcare providers may prescribe medications to mitigate bone loss during chemotherapy. Bisphosphonates, such as alendronate and zoledronic acid, are commonly used to maintain bone density and reduce fracture risk. These medications work by inhibiting osteoclast activity, thereby slowing down bone loss.

5. d. Lifestyle Modifications: Adopting a healthy lifestyle can positively impact bone health during chemotherapy. Avoiding smoking and excessive alcohol consumption, both of which can weaken bones, is crucial. A well-balanced diet rich in fruits, vegetables, whole grains, and lean proteins provides essential nutrients for bone health.

6. e. Regular Monitoring: Regular bone density testing, such as dual-energy X-ray absorptiometry (DXA) scans, can help monitor bone density changes and guide appropriate interventions. Periodic assessments allow healthcare providers to assess the effectiveness of bone health strategies and make adjustments as

## Bone density and fracture risk

Bone density and fracture risk are significant considerations in overall health and well-being. The strength and density of our bones play a crucial role in maintaining mobility and preventing fractures. Various factors, including chemotherapy, can impact bone density and increase the risk of fractures. Below we will explore the relationship between bone density and fracture risk, with a specific focus on how chemotherapy affects these aspects and the implications it carries.

Bone Density and Its Significance:

Bone density refers to the amount of mineral content present in our bones. It reflects the overall strength and density of the skeletal structure. Adequate bone density is vital for maintaining healthy bones and reducing the risk of fractures. Higher bone density signifies stronger bones and a lower risk of fractures, while low bone density indicates weaker bones and an increased risk of fractures.

Factors Affecting Bone Density:

Several factors influence bone density, including genetics, age, sex, hormonal balance, nutrition, physical activity, and certain medical conditions or treatments. Achieving optimal bone density during childhood and adolescence is crucial as it sets the foundation for strong bones throughout life. However, bone density can change over time due to various factors, including hormonal changes, aging, and certain medical interventions such as chemotherapy.

Chemotherapy and Bone Density:

Chemotherapy is a powerful treatment modality used in the management of cancer. While chemotherapy is effective against cancer cells, it can inadvertently impact other parts of the body, including the skeletal system. Certain chemotherapy drugs, such as glucocorticoids and aromatase inhibitors, have been associated with bone loss and decreased bone density.

Glucocorticoids, commonly used in the treatment of inflammatory conditions and some types of cancer, can disrupt the delicate balance of bone remodeling, leading to bone loss. Aromatase inhibitors, frequently prescribed for hormone receptor-positive breast cancer, can cause estrogen deprivation, resulting in accelerated bone loss and increased fracture risk.

Implications of Decreased Bone Density:

Reduced bone density significantly increases the risk of fractures. Fractures can occur from minor falls or trauma that might not typically cause fractures in individuals with normal bone density. Fractures can have severe consequences, leading to pain, limited mobility, decreased quality of life, and increased healthcare costs.

Assessing Bone Density:

Dual-energy X-ray absorptiometry (DXA) scans are commonly used to measure bone density. This non-invasive test provides a T-score, which compares an individual's bone density to that of a healthy young adult. A T-score of -1 or above is considered normal, while a T-score between -1 and -2.5 indicates osteopenia (low bone density), and a T-score of -2.5 or below signifies osteoporosis (significant bone loss).

Strategies to Maintain and Improve Bone Density:

2. a. Nutrition: Adequate nutrition plays a crucial role in maintaining and improving bone density. A diet rich in calcium, vitamin D, and other essential nutrients supports bone health. Calcium sources include dairy products, leafy greens, and fortified foods, while vitamin D can be obtained through sunlight exposure or supplementation.

3. b. Physical Activity: Weight-bearing exercises, such as walking, jogging, dancing, and weightlifting, help promote bone health by stimulating bone remodeling and strengthening bones. Engaging in regular physical activity is important for maintaining bone density and reducing fracture risk.

4. c. Medications: In some cases, healthcare providers may prescribe medications to mitigate bone loss and improve bone density. Bisphosphonates, such as alendronate and risedronate, are commonly prescribed to reduce the risk of fractures and increase bone density. Other medications, including selective estrogen receptor modulators (

## Strategies for maintaining bone health

Bone health is essential for overall well-being and mobility. Individuals undergoing chemotherapy may experience a higher risk of bone loss and fractures due to the treatment's impact on bone density. However, implementing strategies to maintain bone health can help mitigate these risks. Below we will explore various strategies for maintaining bone health, focusing on their relevance and effectiveness in the context of chemotherapy.

Adequate Nutrition:

A well-balanced diet is crucial for maintaining healthy bones. Calcium and vitamin D are two key nutrients necessary for optimal bone health. Calcium-rich foods such as dairy products, leafy greens, and fortified products should be included in the diet. Additionally, vitamin D can be obtained through sun exposure or supplements. It is important for individuals undergoing chemotherapy to discuss their dietary needs with a healthcare provider or registered dietitian to ensure adequate calcium and vitamin D intake.

Weight-Bearing and Resistance Exercises:

Regular physical activity, particularly weight-bearing and resistance exercises, is beneficial for bone health. Weight-bearing exercises include activities where your body supports its weight, such as walking, jogging, dancing, and hiking. These exercises stimulate bone formation and help maintain bone density. Resistance exercises, such as weightlifting or using resistance bands, can also be effective in strengthening muscles and bones. Individuals undergoing chemotherapy should consult with their healthcare team to determine suitable exercise options based on their overall health and treatment plan.

Fall Prevention:

Reducing the risk of falls is crucial for individuals undergoing chemotherapy, as falls can lead to fractures. Implementing preventive measures such as removing hazards from the home environment, using assistive devices (e.g., handrails, grab bars), and wearing appropriate footwear can help minimize the risk of falls. Regular eye check-ups and maintaining proper lighting in the living spaces are also important to enhance safety and prevent accidents.

Medications to Preserve Bone Health:

In some cases, healthcare providers may prescribe medications to minimize bone loss and maintain bone density during chemotherapy. Bisphosphonates, such as alendronate and zoledronic acid, are commonly prescribed to reduce the risk of fractures and increase bone density. These medications work by inhibiting bone breakdown and promoting bone formation. Hormone therapy, such as selective estrogen receptor modulators (SERMs), may also be recommended to preserve bone health in certain cases. It is important to discuss the potential benefits and risks of these medications with the healthcare team.

Smoking Cessation and Alcohol Moderation:

Smoking and excessive alcohol consumption can negatively impact bone health. Smoking has been associated with decreased bone density and increased fracture risk. Alcohol abuse can interfere with the body's ability to absorb calcium and affect bone formation. Individuals undergoing chemotherapy should prioritize smoking cessation and limit alcohol intake to support bone health.

Regular Monitoring and Bone Density Testing:

Regular monitoring of bone health is essential for individuals undergoing chemotherapy. Dual-energy X-ray absorptiometry (DXA) scans can assess bone density and detect any significant changes. Healthcare providers may recommend periodic DXA scans to evaluate bone health and adjust treatment plans accordingly.

Open Communication with Healthcare Providers:

Maintaining open communication with healthcare providers is crucial for individuals undergoing chemotherapy. It is important to discuss any concerns or changes in bone health, such as increased pain, reduced mobility, or fracture incidents. Healthcare providers can provide guidance, offer appropriate interventions, and make necessary adjustments to the treatment plan to support bone health.

Chapter Thirty

# Chemotherapy and Fatigue

Fatigue is a common side effect experienced by many individuals undergoing chemotherapy. It is characterized by a persistent feeling of physical and mental exhaustion that can significantly impact daily functioning and quality of life. Understanding the causes and management strategies for chemotherapy-related fatigue is crucial for individuals undergoing treatment. Below we will explore the relationship between chemotherapy and fatigue, discuss its impact, and provide practical tips for managing and mitigating fatigue during treatment.

Causes of Chemotherapy-Related Fatigue:

Chemotherapy drugs can affect the body in various ways, leading to fatigue. The causes of chemotherapy-related fatigue include:

2. a) Cellular Impact: Chemotherapy drugs target rapidly dividing cells, including healthy cells in the body. This can result in decreased energy production and disruption of normal bodily functions, leading to fatigue.

3. b) Anemia: Chemotherapy can cause a decrease in red blood cell count, leading to anemia. Reduced oxygen-carrying capacity of the blood can result in fatigue and feelings of weakness.

4. c) Sleep Disturbances: Chemotherapy can disrupt sleep patterns, leading to poor sleep quality or insomnia. Lack of restorative sleep can contribute to increased fatigue.

5. d) Emotional and Psychological Factors: Coping with a cancer diagnosis, treatment, and its side effects can cause emotional distress, anxiety, and depression, which can contribute to fatigue.

Impact of Fatigue on Individuals:

Fatigue can significantly impact the daily lives and overall well-being of individuals undergoing chemotherapy. Its effects may include:

6. a) Physical Limitations: Fatigue can lead to reduced physical stamina, making it challenging to perform daily activities, work, or engage in hobbies and social activities.

7. b) Emotional Well-being: Persistent fatigue can contribute to feelings of frustration, irritability, and a sense of loss of control, affecting emotional well-being.

8. c) Cognitive Functioning: Fatigue can impair concentration, memory, and decision-making abilities, making it difficult to perform tasks that require mental focus.

9. d) Quality of Life: Fatigue can diminish the overall quality of life and may affect relationships, work productivity, and the ability to enjoy daily activities.

Strategies for Managing Chemotherapy-Related Fatigue:

While fatigue during chemotherapy can be challenging, there are strategies that can help manage and alleviate its impact. These include:

10. a) Energy Conservation: Prioritize activities and allocate energy to essential tasks. Break tasks into manageable segments and take regular breaks to avoid overexertion.

11. b) Balanced Diet and Hydration: Proper nutrition and hydration are essential for managing fatigue. Eat a well-balanced diet with a variety of nutrients and drink plenty of fluids to maintain hydration.

12. c) Physical Activity: Engage in regular, moderate physical activity as tolerated. Exercise has been shown to reduce fatigue, improve mood, and increase energy levels. Consult with healthcare providers to determine suitable exercise options.

13. d) Sleep Hygiene: Establish a regular sleep routine and create a conducive sleep environment. Avoid caffeine and electronic devices before bed, and practice relaxation techniques to improve sleep quality.

14. e) Emotional Support: Seek emotional support from family, friends, or support groups. Discussing feelings and concerns with a trusted person or mental health professional can help alleviate emotional distress and reduce fatigue.

15. f) Stress Management: Incorporate stress management techniques such as meditation, deep breathing exercises, and mindfulness to reduce stress levels and promote relaxation.

16. g) Medication Management: Speak with healthcare providers about medications or interventions that may help manage fatigue. In some cases, medication adjustments or the use of specific drugs may be recommended.

17. h) Communication with Healthcare Team: Openly communicate with healthcare providers about your fatigue levels and its impact on daily life. They can provide tailored advice, recommend interventions, or adjust treatment plans accordingly.

Support from Loved

## Understanding cancer-related fatigue

Fatigue is a common symptom experienced by individuals undergoing cancer treatment, including chemotherapy. It is characterized by a persistent and overwhelming sense of physical, emotional, and mental exhaustion that can significantly impact a person's quality of life. Understanding the causes, effects, and management strategies for cancer-related fatigue is crucial for individuals undergoing treatment. Below we will explore the concept of cancer-related fatigue, its impact on patients, and discuss strategies for effectively managing and coping with this debilitating symptom.

What is Cancer-Related Fatigue?

Cancer-related fatigue is a type of fatigue that is not relieved by rest and is directly related to cancer and its treatment. It is different from the typical tiredness experienced in everyday life. Cancer-related fatigue can occur at any stage of the disease, but it is particularly common during chemotherapy treatment. It is a multifactorial symptom with various underlying causes, including:

2. a) Treatment Side Effects: Chemotherapy, radiation therapy, and other cancer treatments can directly affect the body's energy levels and contribute to fatigue.

3. b) Anemia: Cancer and its treatments can lead to a decrease in red blood cells, resulting in anemia. Anemia reduces the oxygen-carrying capacity of the blood, leading to fatigue and weakness.

4. c) Inflammation: Cancer triggers an inflammatory response in the body, which can contribute to fatigue.

5. d) Emotional and Psychological Factors: The emotional and psychological burden of a cancer diagnosis, along with anxiety, depression, and stress, can exacerbate fatigue.

Impact of Cancer-Related Fatigue:

Cancer-related fatigue can have a profound impact on all aspects of a person's life, including:

6. a) Physical Functioning: Fatigue can limit a person's ability to engage in daily activities, work, and exercise, resulting in decreased physical functioning and stamina.

7. b) Emotional Well-being: Fatigue can contribute to feelings of frustration, irritability, and depression. It can also affect a person's self-esteem and sense of control over their life.

8. c) Cognitive Functioning: Fatigue can impair memory, concentration, and decision-making abilities, making it challenging to perform tasks that require mental focus.

9. d) Quality of Life: The persistent and overwhelming nature of cancer-related fatigue can significantly diminish a person's overall quality of life. It may lead to social withdrawal, decreased participation in enjoyable activities, and disrupted relationships.

Strategies for Managing Cancer-Related Fatigue:

While cancer-related fatigue can be challenging to manage, there are strategies that can help alleviate its impact and improve overall well-being. These strategies include:

10. a) Energy Conservation: Prioritize and pace activities to conserve energy throughout the day. Break tasks into smaller segments, delegate responsibilities when possible, and ask for help from family and friends.

11. b) Rest and Sleep: Establish a regular sleep routine and create a relaxing sleep environment. Practice good sleep hygiene, such as avoiding caffeine and electronic devices before bedtime, to improve the quality of sleep.

12. c) Physical Activity: Engage in regular, moderate exercise as tolerated. Physical activity can help reduce fatigue, improve mood, and increase energy levels. Consult with healthcare providers to determine suitable exercise options based on individual abilities and treatment regimen.

13. d) Balanced Nutrition: Eat a well-balanced diet that includes a variety of nutrient-rich foods. Consult with a registered dietitian to ensure proper nutrition during treatment and to address any specific dietary needs.

14. e) Emotional Support: Seek emotional support from loved ones, support groups, or mental health professionals. Talking about feelings and concerns can help alleviate emotional distress and reduce fatigue.

15. f) Stress Management: Practice stress management techniques such as meditation, deep breathing exercises, and relaxation techniques. Engaging in activities that promote relaxation and reduce stress can help manage fatigue.

g

## Managing fatigue during treatment

Fatigue is a common and distressing symptom experienced by individuals undergoing chemotherapy. Chemotherapy-related fatigue can significantly impact a person's quality of life, affecting physical, emotional, and cognitive functioning. Managing fatigue effectively is essential to enhance well-being and maintain daily activities during treatment. Below we will explore various strategies and lifestyle modifications that can help individuals better manage fatigue during chemotherapy.

Prioritize Rest and Sleep:

Getting adequate rest and quality sleep is crucial for managing fatigue. Here are some tips to improve rest and sleep:

2. a) Establish a Sleep Routine: Set a regular sleep schedule by going to bed and waking up at the same time each day. Consistency can help regulate the body's internal clock.

3. b) Create a Restful Environment: Make your bedroom conducive to sleep by keeping it dark, quiet, and at a comfortable temperature. Use comfortable bedding and consider using earplugs or eye masks if needed.

4. c) Avoid Stimulants: Limit or avoid caffeine and other stimulants, especially in the evening. Stimulants can interfere with sleep and exacerbate fatigue.

5. d) Practice Relaxation Techniques: Engage in relaxation techniques such as deep breathing exercises, meditation, or listening to calming music before bedtime to promote relaxation and improve sleep quality.

Optimize Physical Activity:

Engaging in regular physical activity can counteract fatigue and improve overall well-being. Here's how to incorporate exercise during chemotherapy:

6. a) Consult with Healthcare Providers: Talk to your healthcare team before starting an exercise program. They can provide guidance on suitable activities and any necessary modifications based on your overall health and treatment plan.

7. b) Start Slowly: Begin with low-impact exercises, such as walking or gentle stretching, and gradually increase the duration and intensity as tol-

erated. Listen to your body and adjust the intensity based on your energy levels.

8. c) Stay Hydrated: Drink plenty of water before, during, and after exercise to prevent dehydration, which can worsen fatigue.

9. d) Choose Enjoyable Activities: Engage in activities that you enjoy and find motivating. This can help you stay consistent and maintain a positive mindset towards exercise.

10. e) Incorporate Rest Days: Allow for regular rest days to give your body time to recover and prevent overexertion.

Conserve Energy:

Conserving energy throughout the day can help manage fatigue and prevent excessive exhaustion. Consider the following strategies:

11. a) Prioritize Tasks: Focus on completing essential tasks first and delegate or postpone non-urgent activities. This way, you can allocate energy to the most important responsibilities.

12. b) Plan Breaks: Schedule short breaks throughout the day to rest and recharge. Use these breaks to engage in relaxation techniques or take a power nap if needed.

13. c) Manage Workload: If you are working or have other commitments, communicate with your employer or school to discuss potential accommodations, such as flexible hours or reduced workload.

14. d) Ask for Help: Don't hesitate to reach out to family, friends, or support services for assistance with daily chores, childcare, or transportation. Accepting help can lighten your load and conserve energy.

Maintain a Nutritious Diet:

Eating a balanced and nutritious diet can provide the necessary energy and nutrients to combat fatigue. Consider the following dietary tips:

15. a) Stay Hydrated: Drink plenty of fluids throughout the day to prevent dehydration, which can contribute to fatigue.

16. b) Balanced Meals: Include a variety of fruits, vegetables, whole grains, lean proteins, and healthy fats in your diet. These provide essential nutrients to support your energy levels and overall health.

17. c) Small, Frequent Meals: Eating smaller, more frequent meals rather than large meals can help prevent energy crashes and promote sustained energy levels.

## Energy conservation and pacing

Fatigue is a common side effect of chemotherapy that can significantly impact the quality of life of individuals undergoing treatment. Chemotherapy-related fatigue can result in decreased energy levels, physical and mental exhaustion, and a reduced ability to engage in daily activities. Managing fatigue effectively requires a multifaceted approach that includes energy conservation and pacing techniques. Below we will explore various strategies to help individuals better manage their energy levels and maintain a balanced and fulfilling life during chemotherapy.

Understand Energy Conservation:

Energy conservation involves using energy wisely to prevent excessive fatigue and preserve energy for essential activities. Here are some key principles of energy conservation:

2. a) Prioritize and Delegate: Identify the most important tasks and focus your energy on completing those first. Delegate non-essential tasks to others or ask for assistance when needed.

3. b) Break Tasks into Smaller Steps: Break down larger tasks into smaller, more manageable steps. This helps prevent overwhelming fatigue and allows for regular rest breaks.

4. c) Use Energy-Saving Techniques: Explore ways to conserve energy during daily activities. For example, sit while performing tasks whenever possible, use assistive devices for support, and arrange your environment to minimize physical exertion.

5. d) Plan and Organize: Create a schedule or plan to optimize your energy use. Group similar activities together and allocate rest periods in between to prevent excessive fatigue.

Practice Pacing:

Pacing involves distributing activities and rest periods throughout the day to maintain a balance between exertion and recovery. Here are some pacing strategies to consider:

6. a) Set Realistic Expectations: Be realistic about what you can accomplish in a day and adjust your expectations accordingly. Recognize that it is okay to pace yourself and take breaks when needed.

7. b) Listen to Your Body: Pay attention to your body's signals and cues. Rest or take breaks at the first signs of fatigue or discomfort, rather than pushing through until exhaustion.

8. c) Use Activity/Rest Cycles: Divide your day into manageable activity and rest periods. Alternate between periods of activity and rest to avoid overexertion and give your body time to recover.

9. d) Gradual Progression: When increasing activity levels, do so gradually. Start with shorter durations or lower intensity and gradually increase as your energy allows.

Optimize Daily Routine:

Modifying your daily routine can help conserve energy and reduce fatigue. Consider the following strategies:

10. a) Plan and Prioritize: Plan your day ahead, considering your energy levels and scheduling important activities during your periods of highest energy.

11. b) Modify Your Environment: Arrange your living or workspace to minimize physical strain. Ensure frequently used items are easily accessible and use tools or aids that can reduce physical effort.

12. c) Efficient Body Mechanics: Learn and practice proper body mechanics to minimize strain and conserve energy when performing tasks. This includes using proper posture, lifting techniques, and body alignment.

13. d) Restorative Breaks: Incorporate short rest breaks or relaxation techniques into your daily routine. These breaks can help rejuvenate your energy and provide mental and physical respite.

Seek Support and Communicate:

Managing fatigue during chemotherapy can be challenging, but you don't have to do it alone. Seek support from healthcare professionals, friends, and family members. Communication is key:

14. a) Talk to Your Healthcare Team: Discuss your fatigue symptoms with your healthcare team. They can provide guidance, assess any underlying causes, and suggest appropriate interventions.

15. b) Educate Your Loved Ones: Help your family and friends understand the impact of fatigue on your daily life. Communicate your needs and limitations, so they can provide appropriate support and assistance.

16. c) Join Support Groups: Connect with support groups or online communities where you can share experiences, gain insights, and receive emotional support from others going through

Chapter Thirty-One

# Chemotherapy and Relationships

Receiving a cancer diagnosis and undergoing chemotherapy treatment can have a significant impact on relationships. The emotional, physical, and practical aspects of chemotherapy can pose unique challenges for individuals and their loved ones. It is crucial to address these challenges openly and support each other throughout the treatment journey. Below we will explore the impact of chemotherapy on relationships and discuss strategies to navigate these challenges while maintaining strong and healthy connections.

Open Communication:

Effective communication is essential during chemotherapy to ensure that everyone's needs and concerns are understood. Here are some communication strategies to consider:

2. a) Share Information: Keep your loved ones informed about your diagnosis, treatment plan, and potential side effects. Provide them with educational materials or involve them in discussions with healthcare professionals to enhance their understanding.

3. b) Express Feelings and Emotions: Encourage open and honest expression of emotions. Both the patient and their loved ones may experience fear, anxiety, or sadness. Sharing these feelings can foster empathy and strengthen the emotional bond.

4. c) Active Listening: Practice active listening to fully understand each other's perspectives. Show empathy and validate each other's emotions, creating a safe space for open dialogue.

5. d) Ask for Support: As the patient, communicate your needs and ask for support when necessary. This may include practical assistance, emotional support, or simply someone to talk to.

Adjusting Roles and Responsibilities:

Chemotherapy treatment may require adjustments to everyday roles and responsibilities within relationships. Here are some considerations:

6. a) Shared Decision-Making: Involve your loved ones in treatment decisions, allowing them to provide input and support. However, ultimately, the final decision should be based on what is best for the patient.

7. b) Redefine Responsibilities: Recognize that the patient may require additional support and assistance during treatment. Redistribute household chores, childcare responsibilities, or financial management to alleviate the patient's burden.

8. c) Flexibility and Adaptation: Understand that the patient's energy levels and abilities may fluctuate during treatment. Remain flexible and willing to adapt plans and expectations to accommodate their needs.

Emotional Support:

Chemotherapy can take an emotional toll on both the patient and their loved ones. It is important to provide and seek emotional support during this challenging time. Consider the following strategies:

9. a) Validate Emotions: Acknowledge and validate each other's emotions. Encourage open conversations and provide a listening ear for the patient's concerns and fears.

10. b) Seek Professional Support: Encourage the patient and their loved ones to seek professional counseling or therapy. A trained therapist can offer guidance and coping strategies to manage the emotional impact of chemotherapy.

11. c) Participate in Support Groups: Joining support groups or engaging with online communities can provide a sense of belonging and connection with others who are going through similar experiences. Sharing experiences, advice, and encouragement can be incredibly helpful.

Intimacy and Sexuality:

Chemotherapy can affect a person's physical and emotional well-being, including intimacy and sexuality. It is important to address these aspects of the relationship with sensitivity and openness:

12. a) Communication and Understanding: Discuss changes in sexual desire, physical limitations, or body image concerns openly and honestly. Explore alternative forms of intimacy and find ways to maintain closeness and connection.

13. b) Seek Professional Guidance: If sexual concerns persist, consider consulting a healthcare professional or a sexual health specialist who can offer guidance and support.

14. c) Emotional Intimacy: Focus on emotional intimacy and find non-sexual ways to connect and support each other. Engage in activities that foster emotional closeness, such as cuddling, holding hands, or engaging in meaningful conversations.

Self-Care and Mutual Support:

Taking care of oneself is crucial when supporting a loved one through chemotherapy. Consider the following strategies:

## The impact of chemotherapy on personal relationships

Chemotherapy is a common treatment for cancer, aiming to eliminate or control the growth of cancer cells. While it is a critical part of cancer care, it can have a profound impact on personal relationships. The physical, emotional, and practical challenges associated with chemotherapy can strain even the strongest of bonds. Below we will explore the impact of chemotherapy on personal relationships and discuss ways to nurture and maintain connections during this challenging time.

Emotional Rollercoaster:

Chemotherapy often triggers a rollercoaster of emotions for both the individual undergoing treatment and their loved ones. It is essential to recognize and address these emotions to maintain healthy relationships:

2. a) Empathy and Understanding: Loved ones should strive to understand and empathize with the emotional journey of the individual undergoing chemotherapy. They may experience fear, anxiety, sadness, or anger. Providing a supportive and non-judgmental environment is crucial.

3. b) Communication: Open and honest communication is key to navigating emotional challenges. Encouraging the individual to express their emotions and actively listening without judgment can foster a deeper connection and provide a sense of comfort and support.

4. c) Patience and Flexibility: Chemotherapy side effects, such as mood swings or irritability, can impact relationships. Being patient and understanding during these moments is vital. Flexibility in plans and expectations can help alleviate stress and maintain a positive atmosphere.

Changes in Roles and Responsibilities:

Chemotherapy can disrupt the normal balance of roles and responsibilities within relationships. It is important to adapt and support each other during this time:

5. a) Redistribution of Tasks: The individual undergoing chemotherapy may have limited energy and physical capabilities. Loved ones can step in and take on additional responsibilities, such as household chores, child-care, or managing finances. Collaboratively redefining roles can alleviate the burden on the patient.

6. b) Teamwork and Collaboration: Emphasize the importance of team-work and collaboration within the relationship. It is a collective effort to navigate through the challenges of chemotherapy. Sharing the load and supporting each other will strengthen the bond between partners, family members, or friends.

7. c) Expressing Appreciation: Recognize and express appreciation for the efforts made by the individual undergoing chemotherapy and their support system. Showing gratitude can foster a sense of validation and promote a positive and supportive environment.

Physical Changes and Intimacy:

Chemotherapy can result in physical changes that may affect personal relationships, including body image, intimacy, and sexual relationships. Nurturing intimacy and fostering open communication can help navigate these changes:

8. a) Body Image: Chemotherapy may cause changes in appearance, such as hair loss, weight fluctuations, or skin problems. Loved ones can provide reassurance, support, and acceptance to help the individual maintain a positive self-image.

9. b) Open Dialogue: Encourage open and honest conversations about physical changes and their impact on intimacy and sexual relationships. Sharing fears, concerns, and desires can foster understanding and facilitate the exploration of new ways to maintain intimacy and connection.

10. c) Seeking Professional Support: If physical changes significantly impact self-esteem or sexual relationships, seeking guidance from healthcare professionals or therapists who specialize in sexual health can be beneficial.

Cultivating Support Networks:

Building a strong support network is essential for both the individual undergoing chemotherapy and their loved ones:

11. a) Support Groups: Encourage the individual to join support groups where they can connect with others going through similar experiences. Support groups provide an outlet for sharing emotions, seeking advice, and finding solace in a community that understands the challenges of chemotherapy.

12. b) Seeking Professional Support: Healthcare professionals, therapists, or counselors can provide guidance, coping strategies, and emotional support to both the individual and their loved ones. Therapy sessions can help individuals process their emotions and provide tools

## Communication and emotional support

Chemotherapy is a challenging and transformative journey for individuals undergoing cancer treatment, as well as for their loved ones. Effective communication and emotional support play a vital role in navigating this journey, fostering understanding, and strengthening relationships. Below we will explore the significance of communication and emotional support during chemotherapy and provide practical strategies to enhance these essential aspects of relationships.

Open and Honest Communication:

Open and honest communication is the foundation of a strong and supportive relationship during chemotherapy. It allows individuals to express their feelings, concerns, and needs while fostering understanding and empathy:

2. a) Active Listening: Active listening involves giving full attention to the person speaking, acknowledging their emotions, and responding in a non-judgmental manner. It is important to create a safe space where the individual undergoing chemotherapy feels comfortable sharing their thoughts and fears.

3. b) Sharing Information: Keeping the lines of communication open regarding treatment plans, side effects, and medical updates is crucial. This helps both the individual and their loved ones stay informed and involved in the journey, allowing them to provide the necessary support.

4. c) Respecting Boundaries: Each person copes with chemotherapy differently, and it is essential to respect boundaries. Some individuals may prefer to discuss their experiences openly, while others may need more privacy. Respecting individual preferences and comfort levels in communication can foster trust and understanding.

Providing Emotional Support:

Chemotherapy often brings about a wide range of emotions for both the individual undergoing treatment and their loved ones. Providing emotional support can help alleviate distress and strengthen the relationship:

5. a) Empathy and Validation: Showing empathy and validating the emotions and experiences of the individual undergoing chemotherapy is crucial. Acknowledge their fears, frustrations, and challenges without minimizing or dismissing their feelings. Empathy creates a safe and nurturing environment for emotional expression.

6. b) Offering Reassurance: Chemotherapy can be physically and emotionally exhausting. Offering reassurance and positive affirmations can provide comfort and uplift the individual's spirits. Simple acts of kindness, such as leaving encouraging notes or small gestures of support, can go a long way in boosting morale.

7. c) Being Present: Being physically and emotionally present is essential during chemotherapy. Attend medical appointments, accompany the individual to treatments, and actively participate in their care. Being present demonstrates love, support, and a willingness to share the journey, fostering a deeper connection.

Effective Problem-Solving:

Chemotherapy can present various challenges that require problem-solving skills to address:

8. a) Collaboration and Decision-Making: Chemotherapy treatment decisions often involve a collaborative effort. Encourage shared decision-making by involving the individual and their loved ones in discussions about treatment options, potential side effects, and supportive care. This collaborative approach strengthens the bond between all parties involved.

9. b) Seeking Professional Guidance: Chemotherapy may bring forth complex medical information and treatment plans. Seeking guidance from healthcare professionals, such as oncologists, nurses, or social workers, can provide clarity and assistance in navigating the treatment process. Pro-

fessional guidance ensures that decisions are well-informed and based on expert advice.

10. c) Problem-Solving Strategies: Together, identify potential challenges and develop problem-solving strategies. This could involve anticipating side effects, managing symptoms, coordinating schedules, or addressing financial concerns. Finding proactive solutions as a team can alleviate stress and promote a sense of control over the situation.

Resilience and Flexibility:

Chemotherapy can be a physically and emotionally demanding journey. Building resilience and maintaining flexibility are vital to supporting the individual undergoing treatment:

11. a) Patience and Understanding: Recognize that the individual may experience physical limitations, fatigue, and mood changes during chemotherapy. Practicing patience and understanding allows for a compassionate response to these challenges, fostering a sense of support and acceptance.

12. b) Flexibility in Plans: Chemotherapy treatment

## Intimacy and sexual health during treatment

Chemotherapy is a crucial aspect of cancer treatment that can have significant effects on various aspects of a person's life, including their intimate relationships and sexual health. It is important to address the topic of intimacy and sexual health during chemotherapy to ensure that individuals and their partners receive the support and information they need. Below we will explore the impact of chemotherapy on intimacy and sexual health, provide factual information, and offer guidance for maintaining a fulfilling and supportive intimate relationship during treatment.

Understanding the Impact of Chemotherapy on Sexual Health:

Chemotherapy can affect sexual health in several ways due to its impact on the body and overall well-being:

2. a) Physical Side Effects: Chemotherapy can cause physical changes such as fatigue, nausea, hair loss, weight changes, and hormonal fluctuations. These side effects can affect body image, self-esteem, and sexual desire.

3. b) Emotional and Psychological Effects: Dealing with a cancer diagnosis and undergoing chemotherapy can result in emotional and psychological distress, including anxiety, depression, and body image concerns. These factors can influence sexual desire, intimacy, and overall sexual well-being.

4. c) Hormonal Changes: Chemotherapy may disrupt hormonal balance, leading to changes in libido, vaginal dryness, and erectile dysfunction. These changes can impact sexual pleasure and satisfaction.

Open Communication and Emotional Support:

Maintaining open communication and providing emotional support are key to navigating intimacy and sexual health during chemotherapy:

5. a) Honest Conversations: Encourage open and honest communication about sexual concerns, desires, and challenges. Create a safe and non-judgmental space where both partners can express their feelings, fears, and needs.

6. b) Seek Professional Guidance: Encourage individuals and their partners to discuss sexual health concerns with healthcare professionals, such as oncologists, nurses, or sexual health specialists. These professionals can provide guidance, address specific concerns, and offer recommendations for managing sexual side effects.

7. c) Emotional Support: Offer emotional support and reassurance to your partner. Be understanding and patient, and validate their feelings and experiences. Assure them that their sexual well-being is important to you and that you are willing to work together to find solutions.

Exploring Alternative Intimate Activities:

During chemotherapy, sexual intimacy may need to be adapted to accommodate physical changes and challenges. Exploring alternative intimate activities can help maintain a fulfilling and connected relationship:

8. a) Emotional Intimacy: Focus on emotional intimacy through cuddling, holding hands, and verbal expressions of love and affection. Emotional closeness can strengthen the bond between partners and foster a sense of connection.

9. b) Non-Sexual Physical Intimacy: Engage in non-sexual physical activities, such as massages or gentle touch, that can provide physical closeness and pleasure without the pressure of sexual performance.

10. c) Intimacy Beyond Intercourse: Recognize that intimacy is not solely dependent on sexual intercourse. Engage in activities that foster connection, such as shared hobbies, quality time together, and open communication.

Managing Physical Side Effects and Seeking Solutions:

Addressing the physical side effects of chemotherapy and seeking appropriate solutions can improve sexual health during treatment:

11. a) Fatigue Management: Fatigue is a common side effect of chemotherapy that can impact sexual desire and energy levels. Manage fatigue by scheduling intimate moments during times of the day when energy levels are higher. Incorporate rest and relaxation techniques to conserve energy.

12. b) Addressing Vaginal Dryness: Vaginal dryness is a common issue for individuals undergoing chemotherapy. Use water-based lubricants to reduce discomfort during sexual activity. Additionally, moisturizers designed for vaginal dryness can be used to alleviate symptoms and improve comfort.

13. c) Erectile Dysfunction Management: For individuals experiencing erectile dysfunction, consult healthcare

Chapter Thirty-Two

# Life After Chemotherapy: Prevention and Wellness

Completing chemotherapy is a significant milestone in a cancer survivor's journey. While it marks the end of a specific treatment phase, it also signifies the beginning of a new chapter focused on prevention and wellness. After chemotherapy, individuals can take proactive steps to promote their overall health, reduce the risk of cancer recurrence, and enhance their well-being. Below we will explore various aspects of life after chemotherapy, emphasizing prevention and wellness strategies that can empower survivors to lead fulfilling and healthy lives.

Embracing a Healthy Lifestyle:

Adopting a healthy lifestyle is crucial for long-term well-being and reducing the risk of cancer recurrence:

2. a) Balanced Nutrition: Focus on a well-rounded diet that includes a variety of fruits, vegetables, whole grains, lean proteins, and healthy fats. Consult with a registered dietitian for personalized dietary recommendations that support immune function and overall health.

3. b) Regular Physical Activity: Engage in regular exercise to promote cardiovascular health, strengthen the immune system, improve energy levels, and enhance overall well-being. Choose activities that align with individual capabilities and preferences, such as walking, swimming, yoga, or strength training.

4. c) Tobacco and Alcohol Avoidance: Quit smoking and limit alcohol consumption to reduce the risk of various cancers and other health complications. Seek support from healthcare professionals or support groups if needed.

Follow-up Care and Medical Monitoring:

Regular follow-up care and medical monitoring are crucial components of post-chemotherapy life:

5. a) Medical Check-ups: Attend scheduled follow-up appointments with healthcare providers to monitor overall health, assess any potential side effects or complications, and discuss ongoing care plans. This may include physical exams, blood tests, imaging scans, and other tests specific to individual needs.

6. b) Survivorship Care Plans: Work with healthcare providers to develop a survivorship care plan that outlines ongoing monitoring, recommended screenings, and long-term follow-up care. This plan serves as a roadmap for maintaining optimal health and addressing any potential late effects or concerns.

7. c) Emotional Support: Seek emotional support through support groups, counseling, or therapy. Dealing with the aftermath of cancer and adjusting to life after chemotherapy can be challenging. Emotional support can help individuals process their experiences, cope with fears or anxieties, and enhance overall well-being.

Cancer Prevention and Risk Reduction:

Taking proactive measures to prevent cancer recurrence and reduce the risk of developing other cancers is essential:

8. a) Regular Screenings: Adhere to recommended cancer screenings, such as mammograms, colonoscopies, and Pap smears, as advised by healthcare professionals. Early detection of any potential recurrence or new cancer is crucial for successful treatment.

9. b) Sun Protection: Protect the skin from harmful UV rays by applying sunscreen with a high SPF, wearing protective clothing, and avoiding excessive sun exposure. Regular skin self-exams can help detect any changes or abnormalities.

10. c) Vaccinations: Stay up-to-date with vaccinations, including those recommended for cancer prevention, such as the HPV vaccine or hepatitis B vaccine.

Emotional Well-being and Mental Health:

Promoting emotional well-being and prioritizing mental health is vital for post-chemotherapy life:

11. a) Self-Care: Engage in activities that promote relaxation, stress reduction, and self-care. This may include practicing mindfulness or meditation, pursuing hobbies, spending time in nature, or engaging in creative outlets.

12. b) Social Support: Maintain and nurture strong social connections. Surrounding oneself with supportive friends, family, or fellow survivors can provide a sense of community, understanding, and encouragement.

13. c) Mental Health Support: Seek professional help if experiencing persistent emotional distress, anxiety, depression, or post-traumatic stress. Mental health professionals can provide guidance, support, and appropriate interventions to promote psychological well-being.

Healthy Relationships and

## Cancer recurrence and prevention strategies

After undergoing chemotherapy, cancer survivors often have concerns about the possibility of cancer recurrence. While the fear of recurrence is understandable, there are several strategies that individuals can embrace to reduce the risk and take control of their health. Below we will explore various aspects of cancer recurrence and prevention strategies, focusing on empowering survivors with knowledge and practical steps to lead a healthy and fulfilling life.

Understanding Cancer Recurrence:

2. a) Definition: Cancer recurrence refers to the return of cancer after a period of remission or successful treatment. It can occur locally (in the same area as the original cancer) or in distant parts of the body.

3. b) Risk Factors: Certain factors may increase the risk of cancer recurrence, including the stage and type of cancer, the effectiveness of the initial treatment, genetics, lifestyle factors, and overall health status.

Maintaining a Healthy Lifestyle:

Adopting a healthy lifestyle is essential for reducing the risk of cancer recurrence and promoting overall well-being:

4. a) Balanced Nutrition: Focus on a diet rich in fruits, vegetables, whole grains, lean proteins, and healthy fats. Limit processed foods, sugary drinks, and red meat. Consult with a registered dietitian for personalized dietary recommendations.

5. b) Regular Physical Activity: Engage in regular exercise to improve overall health and well-being. Aim for at least 150 minutes of moderate-in-

tensity aerobic activity or 75 minutes of vigorous-intensity aerobic activity per week, along with strength-training exercises.

6. c) Smoking Cessation: Quit smoking and avoid exposure to secondhand smoke. Smoking is associated with an increased risk of cancer recurrence and the development of new cancers.

7. d) Alcohol Moderation: Limit alcohol consumption as excessive drinking is linked to an increased risk of cancer recurrence. For individuals who choose to drink, moderation is key, with women advised to limit consumption to one drink per day and men to two drinks per day.

Regular Medical Follow-up:

Regular medical follow-up and surveillance are crucial for detecting any signs of recurrence or new cancers:

8. a) Adherence to Follow-up Appointments: Attend scheduled follow-up appointments with healthcare providers. These appointments may include physical exams, blood tests, imaging scans, and other tests specific to the type of cancer and individual circumstances.

9. b) Communicating with Healthcare Providers: Be proactive in discussing any concerns, symptoms, or changes in health with healthcare providers. Early detection of potential recurrence is key to successful treatment.

10. c) Genetic Testing: Some individuals may benefit from genetic testing to determine their risk of developing certain types of cancer. This information can guide surveillance and prevention strategies.

Managing Stress and Mental Health:

Emotional well-being and stress management play a significant role in overall health and cancer prevention:

11. a) Stress Reduction Techniques: Practice stress reduction techniques such as meditation, deep breathing exercises, yoga, or engaging in hobbies or activities that bring joy and relaxation.

12. b) Support Systems: Maintain a strong support system of friends, family, or support groups who can provide emotional support and understanding.

13. c) Mental Health Support: Seek professional help if experiencing persistent emotional distress, anxiety, or depression. Mental health professionals can provide guidance and support in managing emotional well-being during the post-treatment phase.

Sun Protection and Environmental Factors:

Take precautions to protect yourself from harmful environmental factors:

14. a) Sun Safety: Protect your skin from harmful UV radiation by applying sunscreen with a high SPF, wearing protective clothing, and seeking shade when the sun's rays are strongest.

15. b) Environmental Toxins: Minimize exposure to environmental toxins and pollutants whenever possible. Be aware of potential occupational hazards or harmful substances in your surroundings.

Education and Advocacy:

Stay informed and advocate for your health:

16. a) Stay Updated: Keep abreast of

## Adopting a healthy lifestyle after treatment

After completing chemotherapy treatment, cancer survivors have a unique opportunity to embrace a healthy lifestyle that promotes their overall well-being and reduces the risk of cancer recurrence. By making positive changes in diet, exercise, stress management, and self-care, survivors can take control of their health and create a solid foundation for a fulfilling life. Below we will explore the importance of adopting a healthy lifestyle after treatment and provide practical tips for making sustainable changes.

Nourishing Your Body:

2. a) Balanced Nutrition: Emphasize a balanced diet that includes a variety of fruits, vegetables, whole grains, lean proteins, and healthy fats. Opt for organic and locally sourced foods when possible to reduce exposure to pesticides and additives.

3. b) Portion Control: Pay attention to portion sizes and practice mindful eating. Listen to your body's hunger and fullness cues, and aim for moderation rather than deprivation.

4. c) Hydration: Stay adequately hydrated by drinking plenty of water throughout the day. Limit sugary beverages and alcohol.

5. d) Nutritional Guidance: Consider consulting with a registered dietitian who specializes in oncology to receive personalized dietary recommendations tailored to your specific needs and preferences.

Regular Physical Activity:

6. a) Engage in Exercise: Incorporate regular physical activity into your daily routine. Choose activities you enjoy, such as walking, cycling, swimming, or yoga. Aim for at least 150 minutes of moderate-intensity aerobic exercise or 75 minutes of vigorous-intensity aerobic exercise per week.

7. b) Strength Training: Include strength-training exercises at least two days a week to build muscle strength and improve overall body compo-

sition. This can be done using resistance bands, weights, or bodyweight exercises.

8. c) Outdoor Activities: Take advantage of nature's healing power by engaging in outdoor activities. Spending time in nature has been shown to reduce stress levels and improve overall well-being.

9. d) Seek Professional Guidance: If you are unsure about the right exercise program for your condition or limitations, consult with an exercise specialist or physical therapist who has experience working with cancer survivors.

Managing Stress and Emotional Well-being:

10. a) Stress Reduction Techniques: Incorporate stress reduction techniques into your daily routine. This can include mindfulness meditation, deep breathing exercises, journaling, or engaging in hobbies that bring joy and relaxation.

11. b) Mind-Body Practices: Explore mind-body practices such as yoga, tai chi, or qigong. These practices promote physical and emotional well-being and can help manage stress and anxiety.

12. c) Support Systems: Maintain a strong support system of friends, family, or support groups who understand your journey and can provide emotional support. Share your feelings and concerns with trusted individuals who can lend an empathetic ear.

13. d) Counseling or Therapy: Consider seeking professional counseling or therapy to address any emotional challenges or psychological distress that may arise during the post-treatment phase. Therapy can provide valuable tools and coping strategies to navigate this new chapter of your life.

Quality Sleep:

14. a) Sleep Hygiene: Prioritize quality sleep by establishing a regular sleep schedule, creating a relaxing bedtime routine, and ensuring your sleep environment is conducive to restful sleep.

15. b) Avoid Stimulants: Limit caffeine and electronic device use close to bedtime, as these can interfere with sleep quality.

16. c) Stress Reduction Techniques: Incorporate relaxation techniques, such as deep breathing exercises or meditation, before bedtime to promote a calm and peaceful state of mind.

17. d) Seek Medical Guidance: If you continue to struggle with sleep disturbances, consult with your healthcare provider, who can provide further guidance and support.

Limiting Exposure to Toxins:

18. a) Environmental Toxins: Minimize exposure to harmful toxins and pollutants in your environment. This includes being cautious with household cleaners

## Screening guidelines and long-term care

After completing chemotherapy, cancer survivors need to continue monitoring their health and maintaining regular check-ups to detect any potential cancer recurrence or other long-term health issues. Screening guidelines serve as important tools for early detection, while long-term care ensures ongoing support and optimal health. Below we will explore the significance of screening guidelines and long-term care in relation to chemotherapy, providing valuable insights and recommendations for cancer survivors.

Understanding Screening Guidelines:

2. a) Importance of Regular Screening: Regular screening tests are essential for detecting cancer at its earliest stages or identifying potential complications associated with chemotherapy. These tests can vary depending on the type of cancer, the stage of treatment, and individual factors.

3. b) Collaborative Approach: Effective screening requires a collaborative approach involving healthcare providers, oncologists, and patients. Clear communication between the patient and healthcare team is crucial in determining the appropriate screening tests based on the specific cancer type, treatment history, and individual risk factors.

4. c) Adherence to Screening Guidelines: It is vital for cancer survivors to be aware of and adhere to the recommended screening guidelines. These guidelines outline the recommended frequency and timing of various tests, such as mammograms, colonoscopies, Pap smears, and imaging scans.

Specific Screening Recommendations:

5. a) Breast Cancer: Breast cancer survivors should continue to follow breast cancer screening guidelines, which may include regular clinical breast exams, mammograms, and, in some cases, breast MRI. Self-examination is also encouraged to detect any changes or abnormalities.

6. b) Colorectal Cancer: Colorectal cancer survivors should adhere to regular colonoscopies as recommended by their healthcare provider. These screenings help detect polyps or other abnormalities in the colon or rectum.

7. c) Cervical Cancer: Cervical cancer survivors should continue to follow cervical cancer screening guidelines, which may include Pap smears and HPV testing. These tests help detect any precancerous or cancerous changes in the cervix.

8. d) Other Cancer Types: Depending on the specific cancer type, survivors may require additional screenings such as lung imaging, prostate-specific antigen (PSA) testing for prostate cancer, or imaging scans for lymphoma or leukemia.

Long-Term Care and Follow-Up:

9. a) Survivorship Care Plans: Survivorship care plans are comprehensive documents that outline the individual's treatment history, potential side effects, and recommendations for long-term care. These plans are typically provided by the healthcare team and serve as a guide for the survivor's ongoing care.

10. b) Regular Follow-Up Visits: Regular follow-up visits with healthcare providers are essential for monitoring overall health, addressing concerns, and assessing potential late effects of chemotherapy. These visits may include physical examinations, blood tests, imaging scans, and discussions about emotional well-being.

11. c) Multidisciplinary Approach: Long-term care often involves a multidisciplinary team of healthcare professionals, including primary care physicians, oncologists, specialists, and other supportive care providers. This collaborative approach ensures comprehensive care and addresses the unique needs of cancer survivors.

12. d) Addressing Late Effects: Chemotherapy can have long-term effects on various aspects of health, including the heart, lungs, bones, and cognitive function. Regular monitoring can help detect and manage these late effects promptly.

Lifestyle Factors for Long-Term Health:

13. a) Healthy Diet: Adopting a nutritious diet rich in fruits, vegetables, whole grains, lean proteins, and healthy fats can support overall health and

reduce the risk of chronic diseases. Consultation with a registered dietitian may be helpful for personalized dietary recommendations.

14. b) Physical Activity: Regular exercise has numerous health benefits, including reducing the risk of cancer recurrence, improving cardiovascular health, and enhancing overall well-being. Engage in regular physical activity based on individual capabilities.

*9781776967667*

SD - #0016 - 140926 - C0 - 229/152/21 - PB - 9781776967667 - Matt Lamination